"Drs. Soifer and Himle write with clarity and authority. This book will be of tremendous benefit to those men and women who are burdened by paruresis."

> —Murray B. Stein, M.D., Professor of
> Psychiatry, University of California,
> San Diego

"The authors are to be congratulated: a readable book on this very significant but hidden disorder is long overdue. There is none like it! Their multidimensional discussions of this syndrome and its therapeutic options are excellent. The information they provide has the potential to improve the quality of life for thousands of sufferers."

> —John Marshall, M.D., Professor of
> Psychiatry and Director of the Anxiety
> Disorders Clinic, University of Wisconsin,
> and author, *Social Phobia: From Shyness to
> Stage Fright*

"This is a superb treatment of an embarrassing topic that afflicts millions throughout the world. The authors deserve credit for their efforts to take the mystery out of this common anxiety disorder."

> —Howard Liebgold, M.D., Chief of Kaiser's
> Phobease clinics

"Very comprehensive and well organized. Congratulations on completing such an important work."

> —Carl Robbins, M.S., LCPC, therapist

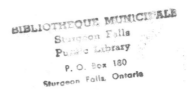

Shy Bladder
SYNDROME

Your Step-by-Step Guide to Overcoming Paruresis

Steven Soifer, M.S.W., Ph.D.

George D. Zgourides, Psy.D.

Joseph Himle, M.S.W., Ph.D.

Nancy L. Pickering

New Harbinger Publications, Inc.

Publisher's Note

This publication is designed to provide accurate and authoritative information in regard to the subject matter covered. It is sold with the understanding that the publisher is not engaged in rendering psychological, financial, legal, or other professional services. If expert assistance or counseling is needed, the services of a competent professional should be sought.

Distributed in the U.S.A. by Publishers Group West; in Canada by Raincoast Books; in Great Britain by Airlift Book Company, Ltd.; in South Africa by Real Books, Ltd.; in Australia by Boobook; and in New Zealand by Tandem Press.

Copyright © 2001 by Steven Soifer, George D. Zgourides, Joseph Himle, and Nancy L. Pickering
New Harbinger Publications, Inc.
5674 Shattuck Avenue
Oakland, CA 94609

Cover design by Lightbourne Images
Edited by Brady Kahn
Text design by Michele Waters

Library of Congress Catalog Card Number: 00-134865
ISBN 1-57224-227-2 Paperback

Printed in the United States of America

New Harbinger Publications' Web site address: www.newharbinger.com

02   01   00

10   9   8   7   6   5   4   3   2   1

First printing

For those who have known the burden of suffering with paruresis.

Contents

Introduction

Imagine this scenario: A man goes to a ball game. He's enjoying the sunshine, the contagious enthusiasm of fellow fans, the hotdogs and the soda. It isn't long before he has to use the men's room. But he cannot urinate in a crowded stadium rest room with its long line of men on the same mission. He reaches the urinal, but the harder he tries, the more it is impossible to go. He needs privacy. Total privacy. Desperate, feeling that his bladder is about to burst, he leaves his friends at the ballpark, drives around until he spots a gas station with an individual toilet and a locked door. He'll be able to urinate there. But he won't be able to get back into the game. Another ruined afternoon—and he can't even tell anyone why.

Millions of Americans suffer from an anxiety problem that few know about and even fewer discuss. This social phobia is *paruresis*, *shy bladder syndrome* (SBS), or *bashful bladder syndrome* (BBS), and it can literally ruin the lives of those who suffer from it. We will use these terms interchangeably throughout the book.

At some point, almost everyone has difficulty urinating, most commonly as a result of medication or while recovering from surgery. But this temporary condition is not bashful bladder syndrome. People who suffer from paruresis, or *paruretics*, almost *always* have trouble using the bathroom if other people are around, even in their own home. Those affected by paruresis describe the feeling as a "freezing" or "locking up" of their bladder, where no amount of will-power affects the ability to urinate. The physical sensation and need to go to the bathroom can be so great it feels as if the bladder might actually burst, but still the paruretic cannot go.

Other than impotence and incontinence, bashful bladder syndrome is perhaps the most embarrassing bodily dysfunction to discuss. For many people, paruresis feels like a deep, dark secret—they do not know why they can't go to the bathroom, but only that they can't. Severe embarrassment prevents most people from discussing the problem, leading them to be extremely isolated and of the mistaken belief that no one else has the problem. In fact, the latest research indicates that approximately 17 million people have difficulty using the restroom away from home. Many suffer from BBS to some degree. Of this number, it is estimated that 1 to 2 million people suffer seriously enough for BBS to significantly interfere with their work, social relationships, travel, and other important activities.

Bashful bladder syndrome does not discriminate. It affects men and women, young and old, straight and gay, and people of all races, ethnicities, and religions. The condition often develops as a result of a traumatic event. The triggering event may be a single episode, which can range from a simple remark ("Will you hurry up and go" spoken to a child going to the bathroom) to sexual abuse. From then on, the paruretic engages in bathroom avoidance behavior, which only perpetuates the problem.

The emotional pain associated with paruresis is severe and crippling. From the father who avoids taking his son to a ball game because he can't use the troughs at the stadium to the mother who doesn't take her daughter clothes shopping because she can't use a department store bathroom, to the executive who loses promotions because he or she cannot travel distances from home to the applicant who loses a job opportunity because he or she can't provide a urine sample for pre-hire drug testing, paruresis destroys lives.

The long-term physical effects of holding one's bladder due to paruresis are not currently known. As yet, no research has been conducted on the subject. What we do know is that not urinating for long periods of time can weaken the elasticity of the bladder, causing less muscle tone. The bladder then needs to empty more frequently, which begins a vicious cycle for the paruretic.

Withholding urine can also cause a buildup of bacteria, increasing the likelihood of urinary tract infections in both men and women. These infections are painful and require medical attention. If the urine is not allowed to be released, the urine can back up into the ureters of the kidneys, which can adversely affect the ureters.

Clearly, it is better to empty the bladder on a regular basis, for physical as well as emotional reasons, making it all the more vital for people with a shy bladder to work toward overcoming the condition.

The good news is that treatment for bashful bladder syndrome is simple: Since a traumatic event triggered the inability to urinate in public, the method to overcome the disorder is to relearn how to urinate in a safe environment. The pace and control of the treatment set forth in this book is in the hands of the paruretic and thus is individualized, which reduces the stress of facing and embracing the process to overcome the phobia. We strongly recommend using a journal when reading the book, to help identify and keep track of those issues that are important, as well as to track your success in overcoming shy bladder syndrome.

Further help can come in the form of support groups, which are springing up in major cities throughout the U.S. and the world. Public awareness of and education about bashful bladder syndrome continues to be at an all-time high, due to recent television, national print, and Internet media exposure, giving hope to those who live with paruresis each day.

This book has nine chapters, providing the reader with crucial information about bashful bladder syndrome: what it is and how to assess whether you or a loved one has it; anecdotes of those who suffer from it; the brain/bladder relationship; the syndrome's causes; self-treatment; controversies surrounding the disorder, including the question of drug testing in the workplace, civil rights, and rest room design; and other bathroom-related phobias.

Paruresis is a devastating affliction, but it does not have to be. Armed with the knowledge and treatment contained in this book, paruretics can overcome this condition and regain control over their lives.

Throughout this book, we will share with you personal stories of people who suffer from shy bladder. These stories are taken from anonymous postings on the International Paruresis Association's (IPA) talk board or from personal communications with the authors, all of whom are on the organization's board of directors. Witness the following description:

> *I am a thirty-one-year-old male who has had this problem for as long as I can remember. It seems as though my case is fairly typical; I can't urinate if I have even the slightest idea that someone might come into the bathroom. I have severe anxiety about it, and it does seem to control my daily movements, thoughts, and behaviors. It doesn't make any sense to me; it isn't rational, but it seems to be the way things are right now.*

Someone may or may not know the cause, but that doesn't really matter. The situation can cause severe depression:

> *I am a twenty-five-year-old male who is having what is supposed to be the best time of my life taken away from me*

by this problem I now know is called paruresis. I have had the problem since I was ten but what difference does it make, since any time with this problem is too long. I thought I was the only one with this problem. It doesn't seem that anyone has found a cure for it. I really can't take this anymore! There are times when I wish I were dead rather than having to deal with this problem. If there is any treatment, please let me know.

But progress is possible, especially if you concertedly work on the problem and apply the techniques outlined in this book. Here is the story of one woman's success:

I think the most incredible experience I have had was a few weeks ago when my husband and I went out for dinner. We went to a restaurant we have been to at least 100 times. I had to go to the bathroom even before we got to the restaurant, which normally produces a lot of anxiety for me. However, not this time. The restaurant was very crowded, and I walked into the bathroom and went. When I got back to the table I realized something, that for as long as we have been going to this restaurant I had never once even walked into the bathroom!

We believe the information and resources found in this book can assist anyone who suffers with this devastating phobia. Knowing you are not alone, knowing you can face this phobia and conquer it, is the first step to living a life free from the interminable, daily prison of paruresis.

CHAPTER ONE

What Is Bashful Bladder Syndrome and How Do You Know You Have It?

A silent medical menace plagues millions of people every day, but no one talks about it. It is a condition informally called *bashful bladder syndrome, shy bladder syndrome, bashful kidneys,* or *pee-phobia.* The official clinical term for the condition is *paruresis.* Regardless of what term is used, BBS is a very real and devastating problem for millions of people who suffer in silence and isolation. Due to the excruciating embarrassment that is part of the syndrome of paruresis, people with BBS are reluctant to discuss it with anyone, including spouse, family, friends, and medical professionals, which only serves to exacerbate the problem.

The purpose of this book is to help you understand the physical and emotional dynamics of paruresis. It will assist you in determining whether or not you have the condition and will provide an overview of both the history of therapeutic approaches to BBS as well as new approaches to treatment. It will also address significant issues that affect people afflicted with paruresis, including the impact of BBS on family members, social situations, relationship difficulties, drug testing in the marketplace, public bathroom design, potential legal ramifications, and accommodations for BBS sufferers in prison.

The time has come to break the cycle of silence and isolation that perpetuates BBS.

What Is Bashful Bladder Syndrome?

It is not uncommon for people to have episodes of trouble using the bathroom at one time or another. Urinary difficulties can arise from a number of medical causes, including medications, strictures or blockages in the urinary system, injury, and disease. However, when a person is physically capable of urinating at home but is unable to urinate anywhere else, the culprit is probably paruresis.

Paruresis is a physiological condition affecting the urinary system that arises from a psychological event. As clinical psychologist and coauthor George Zgourides (1987) explains it:

> After an initial unpleasant experience, the individual antic-ipates difficulty urinating whenever entering a lavatory. Forcible attempts to control the process fail, and associated anxiety with performance reduces the individual's chances of voiding while in a public facility. The paruretic must then adjust to the disorder by voiding as much as possible when at home, restricting the intake of fluids, locating vacant public rest rooms, running the tap, and refusing extended social invitations. (1171–2)

BBS is not limited to public rest rooms. It can also occur in the homes of friends and relatives, or even at the paruretic's own home if visitors are nearby or a family member is "waiting." Typically, paruretics find the home bathroom to be the only truly "safe" toilet—the only one that consistently allows them to void.

Who Has It?

People suffering from BBS frequently believe that they are the only ones in the entire world who have this embarrassing dysfunction. Nothing could be further from the truth. Paruresis may affect as many as *17 million Americans, or about 7 percent of the United States population*, to some degree. Another two million Canadians also suffer from paruresis. It is prevalent among people of all countries, ethnic groups, education levels, and socioeconomic levels—truly a nondiscriminating phobia. People who have BBS are found in every walk of life, including educators, legal professionals, engineers, medical professionals, construction workers, blue collar laborers, and artists. While paruresis occurs among both men and women, 90 percent of people who seek treatment for paruresis are male. We believe, however, that the incidence among the general population is much more evenly distributed.

How to Determine If You Have BBS: A Self-Test

Difficulty passing urine in public rest rooms is not an either/or issue for most. Even among people without bashful bladder syndrome, it is not uncommon to have some hesitancy. Many individuals experience occasional hesitancy both in public rest rooms and at home when attempting to urinate with low urgency, when other people are especially close by, or when trying to urinate quickly while others are waiting. For most individuals, this difficulty is rare and does not lead to a consistent pattern of "freezing up" and avoiding public rest rooms. Paruretics, on the other hand, typically experience increasing trouble urinating in public facilities after initial failures.

Someone with a social phobia is fearful of scrutiny or criticism, but for it to be a true social phobia, this apprehension or fear must lead to a significant interference in the person's daily life. Paruresis is defined as being fearful of passing urine in public rest rooms. In deciding if you feel you meet the criteria for paruresis, you must take into account the degree to which difficulty urinating in public rest rooms disrupts your functioning. For example, occasional hesitancy that doesn't lead to substantial worry or continued difficulty would not constitute a case of paruresis, whereas chronic hesitancy in public facilities that leads to worry, avoidance of social settings, and disruption of normal activities would.

There are various subtypes of paruresis. The most severe group includes people who cannot urinate under any circumstances away from home. At this level of severity, paruretics may make arrangements to live near work, work inside the home, and limit outings to a few hours at a time. Individuals with this level of hesitancy generally avoid fluids and develop distended bladders from holding urine, both of which are physically unhealthy as well as psychologically harmful.

In men's rest rooms, traditionally there are stalls that contain commodes surrounded by walls and a door that locks, and urinals. The urinal setup may be comprised of either a series of low bowl urinals, or wall urinals that protrude in varying degrees from the wall. An important issue for male paruretics is whether or not there are partitions between the urinals.

7

Thankfully, most paruretics can urinate in public rest rooms under some conditions, depending on the configuration of the rest room. For example, some paruretics can urinate using a stall as long as no one is present in the rest room and no one is approaching from the outside. Another subgroup can urinate using a stall when others are present. Still others can urinate using a stall when other people are present, but cannot do the same at a urinal. Yet another subgroup can urinate at a urinal if there are partitions and no one is standing right next to them. Noise level, the size of the rest room, and the level of urgency are variables that most influence a paruretic's ability to urinate in public.

The following self-test is designed to help you assess whether you meet the criteria for bashful bladder syndrome:

1. Do you have a marked and persistent fear using public rest rooms while others are present?

   _____ Yes _____ No

2. Do you experience problems starting your urine in public facilities when others are present?

   _____ Yes _____ No

3. Do you worry about what other people are thinking when you are trying to urinate?

   _____ Yes _____ No

4. Are you able to urinate at home when you can't do so away from home?

   _____ Yes _____ No

5. Are you concerned about being humiliated or embarrassed by problems passing urine?

   _____ Yes _____ No

6. Does attempting to urinate in public rest rooms always, or almost always, provoke anxiety?

   _____ Yes _____ No

7. Does the fear of using public rest rooms seem excessive or unreasonable to you?

   _____ Yes _____ No

8. Do you avoid urinating in public rest rooms and/or do you endure the public rest room situation with intense anxiety or distress?

_____ Yes _____ No

9. Does your avoidance of public rest rooms or anxiety and distress about using public rest rooms interfere significantly with your job, social activities, relationships?

_____ Yes _____ No

10. Has your doctor ruled out a physical cause for your difficulty urinating in public rest rooms?

_____ Yes _____ No

If you answered *yes* to most of the above questions in our paruresis diagnosis inventory, you meet the criteria for bashful bladder syndrome. The more positive responses you have, the more severe your condition probably is. If you answered *yes* to several of the above questions, you may or may not have bashful bladder syndrome. Be sure to check with a trained clinical professional.

When and Where It All Starts

While not every paruretic reports knowledge and/or awareness of an initial triggering experience, many BBS sufferers can point to a traumatic event or circumstance that set the BBS in motion. Although some paruretics report having urination difficulties as young as four and five years of age, for many paruretics the triggering event occurs in early adolescence, usually in a bathroom environment. The triggering event "locks in" the difficulty of being able to void in public. Since this kind of event happens to many people in adolescence, and not everyone develops BBS, it may be that there is a biological propensity and/or psychological sensitivity toward paruresis. It is also possible that people who develop paruresis are prone to experience a single learning event, so that one bad experience will beget a lifetime pattern of BBS.

Coauthor Steve Soifer shares his story:

As a child of eleven or twelve, I was labeled by an elementary school teacher as a "girl," due to an unfortunate situation in the classroom. From that day forward, most of the boys in the class teased me unmercifully. Then one day, I was trying to

> *use one of the urinals in the boys' room and several other*
> *boys began to harass me, demanding to see my "equipment."*
> *Seeking privacy, I went into a bathroom stall. Unrelenting, the*
> *other boys tried to break down the door and climb over it, as*
> *they continued their taunts. From that day forward, I have*
> *suffered from BBS.*

It is important to note that in the medical literature written on paruresis over the years, a number of different hypotheses as to its cause have been presented. These have included: sexual abuse, the inability to express hostility, an internalized wish for punishment, an unconscious association of urination with sexuality, fright or embarrassment, anxiety arousal caused by interpersonal space invasion, biochemical imbalances in the brain, obsessive-compulsive disorder, cultural variables (for example, being raised in a puritanical household), vicarious learning (either through direct observation or stories being told to those who develop paruresis), and instructions by significant others to be concerned about one's bodily functions. (See appendix A.)

As more people with BBS have come forward, a different causal picture has begun to emerge. Though there may be instances of BBS having been triggered by the variables listed above, increasingly paruretics report a history that is inconsistent with these profiles. This may explain why traditional talk therapies have been so unsuccessful in treating those affected with paruresis. Treatment modalities that focus on reconditioning the behavior appear to be more successful.

Case studies of people who have paruresis are invaluable, but the reluctance of most people who experience paruresis to speak about the condition has added to a near vacuum of information. If more people suffering from BBS would come forward, and were met by a better informed medical community, the information gained would significantly aid the search for more effective treatments. More information would also help researchers identify triggering events and environments, and enable them to educate the general public on how to avoid creating those situations that appear to start the cycle of paruresis.

Paruresis—A Social Phobia

For all that we *don't* know about paruresis, we *do* know that paruresis is a social phobia, which is a mental condition popularly known as "stage fright." According to the *Diagnostic and Statistical Manual of*

Mental Disorders (DSM) IV of the American Psychiatric Association (1994), a social phobia (Code 300.23) is a strong fear of embarrassment or humiliation in a social setting and the fear that others will judge one's performance. With social phobias, there is a lot of anxiety associated by the thought of, or actually being exposed to, the dreaded situation. Social phobics realize that their fear response is greatly exaggerated in comparison to the situation. But despite this self-awareness, they continue to avoid triggering settings (for paruretics, a bathroom setting), often going to great lengths to do so.

Very few books and little professional literature dealing with social phobias mention paruresis. The *DSM-IV* and the National Institute of Mental Health (NIMH) (1994) social phobia pamphlet both include paruresis as a type of social phobia. In his popular book *Social Phobia: From Shyness to Stage Fright*, Marshall (1994) devotes three pages to what he calls "Bashful Bladder," stating that "it is well known to our anxiety patients." Markway et al. (1992) in *Dying of Embarrassment: Help for Social Anxiety and Phobia*, give it a page. And in Fezler's (1989) *Creative Imagery: How to Visualize in All Five Senses*, the author gives an example of how one of his clients who had paruresis was "cured" through visualization techniques. Finally, while Bourne's (1995) *The Anxiety and Phobia Workbook* only mentions paruresis in passing, the exercises in that book have been helpful for a number of paruretics.

Triggering Events

Paruretics most commonly refer to three categories, or parameters, that they consider triggering settings. First, other people present in the rest room can trigger BBS, with strangers usually leading to greater inhibition than friends or relatives. Second, proximity (or personal closeness) plays a role in triggering the problem. Proximity for the paruretic is both physical, involving the relative nearness of others in or near the rest room, as well as psychological, involving the need for privacy in order to urinate. For example, most paruretics cannot urinate in a stall toilet if the door is missing. They feel embarrassed that their personal space is being invaded visually. And third, temporary psychological states, especially anxiety, anger, and fear, can interfere with urination. Social phobics who are overly sensitive about the sounds and smells that they make while urinating are usually fearful of being criticized for such, which often leads to the inability to initiate urine. Excessive emotional states may also explain why attempts to urinate under favorable conditions may be unsuccessful when the individual is overly excited, angry, or pressured to hurry.

Like other social phobics who fear public speaking, writing, or blushing in public, paruretics are unusually shy and reserved when it comes to urinating, even though in all other aspects of their personality they may or may not be shy at all. The paruretic fears being scrutinized or criticized by others when "performing" in public. Thus, for paruretics, the public rest room is the "stage" and the performance is the act of urinating on demand. As one person remarked:

> I know it sounds crazy, but when I am in the rest room and someone comes in, I feel like that person's focus is on me and what I am doing, even though they obviously came into the rest room to tend to their own physical needs. It feels like they are thinking about what I am doing, how long I am taking, how much I am going, and whether or not what I am doing is "normal." It makes me very self-conscious, and I can feel myself freeze up. Then, I just can't go, because I'm worrying about whether or not I measure up to what they think is okay, even though the truth is, they probably never even noticed I was there.

BBS As a Specific vs. General Social Phobia

BBS is a specific form of social phobia. Some paruretics are only afraid of situations in which they would need to use a rest room with other people around; others are afraid of many, if not all, social situations. While social phobias are generally more prevalent among women, in terms of the clinical population, paruresis appears to be more common among men (in a ratio of 9:1). There also appears to be a higher incidence of social phobia in general, and paruresis in particular, among direct biological relatives, such as siblings. (The relationship between social phobia, the brain and urination is discussed in Chapter 2.)

People with social phobia also may experience, according to *DSM-IV*, being very sensitive to criticism, perceived or real; negative judgment by others, or not being accepted by others; feelings of non-assertion, poor self-esteem, and inferiority; and "fear [of the] indirect evaluation of others" (APA 1994, 413).

Paruretics can readily identify with these sorts of experiences and feelings but the performance anxiety associated with BBS specifically centers on initiating and maintaining urine flow in public facilities when people are present or might walk in. Paruretics fear that others who see or hear them urinating will criticize or judge them negatively. They worry about looking weak, "crazy," or stupid. They fear producing objectionable odors or sounds while using the toilet. They dread being embarrassed. They hate rejection.

Experts generally agree that social phobias, including BBS, are not rooted in physical dysfunction, but are instead psychological disorders generated by irrational worry over "what others might think" which may then lead to the manifestation of physical symptoms.

How Paruretics Cope—Isolation and Avoidance

Urinating is a normal body function experienced on a daily basis by everyone. There is simply no way to avoid the need to eliminate fluid waste materials from the body. Urinating is such a natural function that most people take the ability to relieve themselves on demand for granted. Conversely, the inability to perform such a basic human task on demand results in tremendous, even overwhelming, feelings of shame and embarrassment. Shame, embarrassment, isolation, and avoidance surrounding the act of urination are all by-products of bashful bladder syndrome. These negative feelings prevent paruretics from both speaking about the problem and seeking treatment, leading to isolation, and setting into motion a spiral of secrecy and avoidance that further compounds the condition.

As might be expected, paruretics become very adept at developing avoidance behaviors and coping mechanisms to deal with the problem. Typical behaviors include holding urine for inordinate amounts of time; depriving oneself of fluids to reduce the need to urinate; depriving oneself of alcohol intake due to its diuretic effect; attending only those public places such as restaurants and movie theaters that are close to home; avoiding travel (including driving distances as well as air travel); avoiding sports stadiums (where bathroom facilities are a paruretic's worst nightmare); and plotting out activities according to where the closest "safe" bathroom facility (such as a one-room bathroom of a service station) is located.

Avoiding social situations, dodging friends or coworkers, and revolving one's life around the location of rest rooms is an exhaustive and consuming response to a shame-filled reality of day-to-day living in the life of the paruretic. The intricate avoidance behaviors that a paruretic develops over the years only appear to yield coping success. Altering your life to accommodate the condition is, at best, merely that—an accommodation. The unfounded belief that no one else suffers from this problem further conspires to keep paruretics in an emotional prison, where there appears to be no real alternative to the paruretic dance of secrecy and avoidance.

Witness this story:

I'm thirty-nine years old [and] have three children and a wife.... I've never been on a vacation in my life, never really going anywhere much. My wife and I [have] been out maybe three times all together in eighteen years of marriage. Well, [it] looks like I may lose her soon; she can't stand me anymore. She keeps wanting me to take her out to dinner, or to the movies.... It's so bad I get very mad and say some things I don't mean ... but I've not been [able to tell her] why.

And another story:

I can remember specific instances in grade school—say, second grade or so—when I had difficulty in a crowded bathroom. This was public knowledge, and I was teased about it.... Forget about going to a bar for a quick drink. Traveling is bad. Sometimes I just suffer.... Driving is the worst because it takes longer to get from A to B and roadside stops are often unsuccessful. This is one of the reasons I hate parties, and never go to big events like ball games and so on, even though I enjoy them. My wife knows about this, but only after years of hiding it.

Ironically, the more paruretics hide the problem, the more the condition is perpetuated. Self-imposed secrecy fuels the avoidance dynamics of the phobia. Conversely, when paruretics begin to tell family and loved ones of their "embarrassing little secret" (as one paruretic called it), the symptoms have been known to diminish. Talking to someone close begins the process of breaking the secret/isolation/avoidance black hole spiral. (The impact of paruresis on family and loved ones is discussed in greater detail in chapter 7.)

Degrees of Intensity—Mild to Severe

As we indicated earlier, BBS ranges in intensity from mild to severe. In mild cases, paruretics can use public facilities under certain circumstances, such as when alone in a public rest room. In severe cases, paruretics may only be able to urinate when alone at home.

The degree of BBS hesitancy ranges from a momentary delay in starting urination to the total inability to institute a urine stream. There is currently no research available to discern what percentage of BBS sufferers fall into which category. However, anecdotal evidence suggests that approximately 10 percent of paruretics, or 1 to 2 million people, suffer from severe paruresis to the degree that their lives are adversely affected and controlled by it on a daily basis.

Most paruretics describe the need for a personal "comfort threshold" in order to urinate, whether in public facilities or at home. When this comfort threshold is eclipsed by a negative circumstance (such as noise, odor, lack of privacy, other people talking while in the rest room), BBS is triggered and prevents them from urinating. The comfort threshold varies among paruretics, according to the severity of the condition. For example, a paruretic with a mild case of BBS might be able to successfully urinate while in an enclosed stall if someone else in the rest room is quietly at the other end of the room, while paruretics with severe BBS may not be able to urinate at all unless no one else is present within their sight or hearing. (The dynamics of this comfort threshold are more thoroughly discussed in chapter 3.)

Lack of an Informed Medical and Mental Health Community

Within the medical and mental health communities, there is an incredible lack of information about and sensitivity to BBS, which only adds to the problem. For those paruretics who gather the courage to turn to a doctor or therapist for help, the response is more often than not (1) the problem is all in their heads and therefore can be controlled through "willing" themselves to go; (2) everyone has the problem once in a while, so "get over it"; or (3) stop worrying about it—if you have to go badly enough, you will.

Said one person:

I've had this problem for about thirty-five years, and have been treated by several professionals, unfortunately with little success.

Another person writes:

I'm a twenty-six-year-old male and have had this problem since I was sixteen. I went to see a couple of urologists first, one of which had never heard of it; the second used the expression "nervous bladder," said I was okay physically, and suggested I see a psychiatrist. I've been seeing a couple of psychiatrists now for about a year, and am now getting kind of depressed because nothing has helped in the least. . . . I guess you can tell I'm bitter at times because so much of my life has been wasted.

Doctors and therapists who are consulted by BBS clients often don't know what to do.

I've talked to two medical doctors and a few counselors about this once I worked up the nerve. In the case of the M.D.s, both times I went through an embarrassing prostate examination, [was] declared healthy, and sent on my way. . . . As for the counselors, they seemed to skirt around the issue, either not understanding what a severe problem it was for me or simply not understanding the problem at all.

The lack of validation from medical providers further deepens the despair of paruretics and fuels their decision not to talk about the problem with others. While such unsympathetic responses from the medical community are born of ignorance, not malice, they are also fed by the cloak of secrecy that paruretics invoke as a result of their shame. It is a vicious cycle. Heightened awareness and discourse among both the medical community *and* the general public is *crucial* to gain understanding, insight, and ultimately the use of successful treatment modalities for the plethora of people who suffer daily from this social phobia.

Other Fears and Urination

To help assess whether you have BBS, it is important to note that there are other reasons besides BBS that people fear public rest rooms. The most common syndromes other than BBS where fear of public rest rooms may be present are:

Obsessive-Compulsive Disorder (OCD)

OCD is a condition where two problems are usually present: repetitive thoughts or worries known as *obsessions,* and repetitive behaviors known as *compulsions.* Obsessions are often difficult to control and cause severe anxiety, while compulsions are usually employed to reduce obsessive thinking and the anxiety that accompanies it. Compulsions are usually performed according to strict rules and often have to be repeated again and again in order to produce relief.

Among the most common obsessions are those that relate to fears of dirt, germs, and contamination. People with contamination obsessions usually respond to these thoughts by avoiding places that are "contaminated," such as public rest rooms. Contamination from human waste often looms large in their imagination. The main issue for avoiding public rest rooms for OCD sufferers is *not* the fear of urinating in front of others but the fear of getting ill or very dirty by coming in contact with public rest room surfaces such as door handles, flusher handles, toilet seats, and sink surfaces.

Someone with OCD may have difficulty urinating in public, because of a fear of urine hitting the urinal or toilet, mixing with urine/feces from others, and then splashing back onto the person with OCD. Many people with OCD spend as little time in public rest rooms as a severely impaired paruretic.

Agoraphobia and Panic Attacks

Agoraphobia is a condition that involves fear and avoidance of situations from which escape would be difficult or help unavailable in case of a panic attack. Panic attacks are anxiety episodes that occur suddenly, unexpectedly, and involve several physical and emotional symptoms. Typical symptoms of a panic attack are shortness of breath, heart palpitations, sweating, trembling, dizziness, feelings of unreality, depersonalization, and fears of dying or losing control. Agoraphobics often fear traveling far from home, entering grocery or department stores, visiting theaters or attending sporting events, and driving in an automobile. When agoraphobics enter these situations, they often feel the need to exit immediately.

People suffering from agoraphobia and panic attacks may fear entering public rest rooms because of concerns about not being able to leave the rest room quickly in order to get help, or not being able to escape to a place of safety in case of a panic attack. Their fear does not involve the fear of urinating in front of others as BBS does. Obviously, urinating or having a bowel movement takes some time to complete, which may cause anxiety for someone anticipating the need for a quick exit. Difficulties with public rest rooms are compounded for agoraphobics because rest rooms are frequently located far within a store or public building, making escape seem all the more problematic.

Claustrophobia

People who have a fear of closed-in places suffer from claustrophobia. Since many public rest rooms are small and lack windows, the claustrophobic may fear the public rest room. Claustrophobics may fear using bathroom stalls because of the perception of being closed in. Crowded rest rooms may also be of concern to claustrophobics due to the perception of long lines and people blocking the exits.

Fear of Crime

Some people fear using public rest rooms because of concerns about crime. In the past, they may have experienced unwanted sexual advances, physical assault, or robbery, or witnessed drug abuse, drug trafficking, or other criminal activity in a public restroom. People who fear crime in public rest rooms often feel that they are especially vulnerable when urinating or defecating. These concerns may result in a pattern of rest room avoidance similar to that of paruretics.

Summary

If being able to urinate any place other than home is difficult or impossible for you, and medical causes have been ruled out; if your life revolves around making daily decisions based on the location or proximity of "safe" rest rooms; and if you feel embarrassed, ashamed, and isolated about your inability to urinate on demand, then you probably have bashful bladder syndrome.

The good news is, once the problem is identified, the process for seeking successful treatment naturally follows.

CHAPTER TWO

The Brain, Bladder, and Urination: Working in Harmony, but Not Always

As we discussed in chapter 1, often BBS is a physiological condition affecting the urinary system that arises from a psychological event. In order to understand the dynamics of the phobia, we must first look at both the psychological causes and physical symptoms of the condition.

The Brain and Urination

Psychologists, psychiatrists, social workers, and other mental health professionals have traditionally labeled physical symptoms arising from a psychological event as *psychogenic, psychosomatic,* or *hysterical conversion.* This means that the physical problems are real, but the cause is mental rather than physical. Some common examples of psychogenic symptoms are headaches or stomach problems arising from situations such as stress at work, or a houseful of unexpected guests. Blindness or limb paralysis, sometimes observed in people after exceptional trauma like war or rape, are more extreme examples of the same process. Whatever the situation, it is important to remember is that the body and mind are so intimately related that the proverbial "mind-body connection" is a fact of everyday life for everyone.

Recent public focus on the effects of stress, the need for exercise, and the benefits of relaxation techniques all underscore an evolving awareness of and healthier attitude toward the mind-body connection. What many people do not realize, however, is just *how* finely attuned the human body and mind are and how the mind can influence the body in unexpected ways. The power of suggestion, Pavlovian responses, and the placebo effect are all examples of this strong connection.

Why Paruretics Cannot Force Themselves to Pee

BBS is characterized by the bodily symptom of not being able to urinate "at will," a symptom that is psychologically generated. The body's bladder responds to what the mind is telling it to do. Thus the problem of BBS is primarily mental, not physical—as opposed to bladder disorders due to physical disease, obstruction, or other conditions such as bladder injury, urethral strictures, cancer, or benign prostatic hyperplasia (an "enlarged prostate"). This does not mean that paruretics can consciously dictate mental directions to the body to urinate on demand. Quite the contrary. The act of urination is a complex physiological process which the mind subconsciously influences:

> *I know this thing is all in my head, but I still can't help but get mad at my bladder for not doing what I tell it to do. How do I know it's a head thing? Because I don't have any trouble going when I'm at home. I'm as relaxed as can be. But when I'm out—at the mall or at a movie theater—it's an entirely different story. My mind seems to be on "hyper-alert" or something. No matter how hard I try, I can't calm things down enough to start peeing.*

You may wonder why the brain would prevent any of us from urinating in public places. The reasons vary among individuals and situations, but BBS is ultimately the result of the psychological processes of *sensation*, *perception*, and *interpretation*.

Sensation, Perception, and Interpretation

Much of what and how we perceive events in the external world depends on our internal world—our personality, temperament, preferences, biases, influences, and so on. That is why our reactions to the same activity or event can differ so dramatically. For instance, one person might not have "hang-ups" about appearing nude in front of others, while another person might be exceptionally modest and refuse to undress in public locker rooms.

Not all perception occurs on a conscious level. In fact, most of the information we receive from the world enters the mind below our levels of awareness. We are not alert to everything going on in our minds, nor can we control all that goes on in our minds. The majority of our mental processes are actually involuntary, meaning they are not under our conscious control.

Since the world is full of things to enjoy as well as things to avoid, the brain must determine what to embrace versus what to reject. In order to do this, the brain first takes in information and then decides what is safe and what is not. Psychologists tell us that the two mental processes human brains require to do this are sensation and perception.

Sensation

Sensation is the ability to respond to sensory information in the external world. Our sensory organs contain *sensory receptors*. The sensory receptors' job is to act like a translator between the environment and the brain. The sensory receptors receive information from the environment and then translate that information into nervous system signals that the brain can perceive and interpret. The human body accomplishes this by the use of the five senses: Sight, sound, smell, taste, and touch.

Perception

Perception is the mental process whereby the human brain "makes sense" of the sensory information collected by the sensory organs. It is as if the sensory organs bring all the information to the brain and say, "Here you go, here are the sights and sounds I took in from the environment. It's all yours." Perception then kicks in to organize the information and to make sense of it. Without perception, the sensory information would be a meaningless swirl of colors, sights, and sounds.

Interpretation

Once the brain perceives the information, it then interprets that information in order to make decisions. For example, when something is "good" (such as eating a chocolate sundae) or "safe" (such as getting into your car), our brains are making *interpretations* based on perceptions of the environment.

One of the strongest influences on those interpretations is *past experience*. A typical sensation-perception-interpretation process is dramatized in the following example: A parent warns a young child not to touch the stove because it is hot. The child touches the stove anyway. When the child's hand comes in contact with the hot stove, the heat is received by the sensory receptors and sends that information to the brain (sensation). The brain perceives the information and recognizes pain and threat (perception). The brain then concludes that touching the hot stove is a threatening experience to the body that will produce pain (interpretation), an experience that will deter the child from touching the hot stove again.

Let's relate this process to BBS: A traumatic occasion of urinating in a public rest room is taken in by the sensory receptors and is sent to the brain (sensation), which perceives the event as painful and a threat (perception). The brain then concludes that going into a public rest room and urinating is painful and a threat (interpretation), which will deter the BBS sufferer from being able to urinate in a public rest room again. The conscious mind is not aware of this process and cannot override it by "wanting" to go. Thus, it is the subconscious perception of a threat that triggers the physical inability to urinate, despite the conscious desire to do so. The subconscious, in an attempt to "protect" the BBS sufferer from the perceived threat of a public rest room, shuts down the urinary system, and overrides the conscious desire to urinate.

Psychological Triggers of Bashful Bladder Syndrome

As we discussed in chapter 1, some of the common triggers causing the brain to block the process of urination include anxiety, anger, sensitivity to scrutiny and criticism, proximity to others, invasion of "personal space," presence of strangers, lack of visual or auditory privacy, lack of suitable partitioning, and sensitivity to odors and noises. If you are prone to this form of social phobia, these conditions or circumstances trigger your brain—whether consciously or unconsciously—to perceive the public rest room or the presence of others in the rest room as a threat.

A typical BBS woman remarks:

> *In elementary school the inability to urinate in public places, or if I thought someone was in hearing distance, was a major problem. I almost never went during school hours and once held my bladder for forty-eight hours during a Girl Scout trip when I was unable to find an empty rest room. My family often referred to me as the "iron bladder." . . . There are times, occasionally, when it just doesn't work. Particularly if I'm in a public rest room and there is a line. The pressure of knowing someone is waiting compounded with the knowledge that many people can hear me is very hard to overcome.*

The threat may be embarrassment (e.g., humiliation at being seen in a public rest room), scrutiny (e.g., criticism for making "objectionable" odors and/or sounds), physical danger (fear of being attacked or castrated), or even sexual arousal (conflicts over homosexual desires), to name only a few possibilities. Remember, the brain's perception of the threat need not be conscious, even though its response manifests as a very real reaction in the person.

The Physiological Structure of the Brain

To understand the interaction between the mind and body, it is important to review the basic physiological structure of the brain.

The human brain and spinal cord make up the *central nervous system*, which coordinates with the *peripheral nervous system* to send and receive *neural signals*, or signals relating to the senses, from the brain to the rest of the body, and vice versa. The peripheral nervous system further divides into the *somatic system* and the *autonomic system*.

The Somatic System

The somatic system is responsible for neural transmission (or communication) occurring between the brain and the voluntary muscles of the body. Simply put, the somatic system allows us to carry out a decision to move a hand, lift a leg, or wiggle our toes.

The Autonomic System

In contrast, the autonomic system is responsible for neural transmission occurring between the brain and the *involuntary* muscles, glands, and systems of the body. For example, the autonomic system is responsible for maintaining heart rhythm, respiration while we are awake and asleep, and food passing through our digestive tracts. If it weren't for the autonomic system, we would have to consciously make our hearts beat, breathing continue, and food digest.

The autonomic system further divides into two additional systems, the *sympathetic system* and the *parasympathetic system*.

The Sympathetic System

The sympathetic system mobilizes the body for physical action. In particular, it causes our pupils to dilate, heartbeat and respiration rates to increase, and digestion and urine volume to decrease, and it causes the urinary bladder wall to relax, which prevents urination. The sympathetic system is also responsible for the *fight or flight* response, a mobilization of the body's various systems to provide us with the ability to either battle a threat or run from it. The entire body is on high alert, ready for immediate action.

The Parasympathetic System

The parasympathetic system quiets the body for rest and energy conservation. It causes the pupils to constrict, heartbeat and respiration rates to decrease, digestion and urine volume to increase, and the urinary bladder wall to contract, which facilitates urination.

BBS primarily involves the autonomic nervous system, and in particular the sympathetic system. When the brain responds to an actual or perceived threat, the autonomic nervous system responds with an increase of sympathetic system activity. (Remember, the sympathetic system physically gears up the body so it can handle a threat.) When people with BBS enter a public rest room, their brains perceive a threat. The sympathetic system is triggered, prompting them to take flight for safety—to leave the rest room for the safety of their bathroom at home.

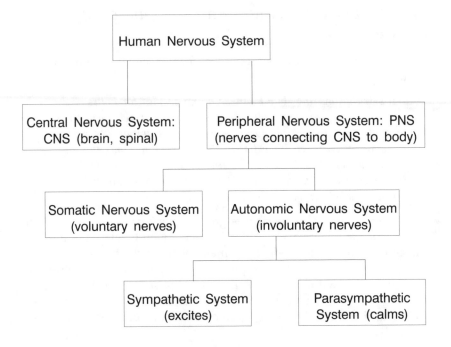

Figure 2.1   The Human Nervous System

What a Paruretic Feels in a Public Rest Room

A paruretic may experience certain physical symptoms as a result of the triggering of the sympathetic system when attempting to urinate in a public rest room. These include the inability to initiate urination, an accelerated heart rate, an increased breathing rate, an increased release of epinephrine by the adrenal glands, blushing, sweating, and increased salivation.

These responses are a result of the autonomic nervous system and are *involuntary*. The sympathetic system is in control, "protecting" the paruretic from the "threat" of a public rest room, and it will not allow the paruretic to urinate until he or she is in a "safe" environment, which is usually at home. The conscious mind and will simply cannot override the mandate of the sympathetic system's flight response.

The Bladder—Why Paruretics Physically Can't Urinate

A typical remark by "Bob," a former client of one of the coauthors:

> *It's truly amazing, but I can be dying to piss for hours. I went twenty-six hours once because I couldn't get away from people on a trip. Anyway, as soon as the situation becomes favorable, I can go immediately. But until I'm alone, nothing will happen. People just don't understand what it's like. I especially like the people who tell me to drink so much beer until I won't be able to hold it. Right!*

Even when Bob experiences great urinary urgency, his bladder won't contract and his bladder's valves won't relax because of increased adrenaline. Indeed, a malevolent cycle takes over. The more Bob unsuccessfully attempts to urinate and the more he tries to force urination without success, the more his brain perceives a threat and physiologically blocks the process. Yet, as soon as Bob locates an isolated toilet, his brain no longer perceives a threat, and he urinates instantly.

How the Process of Urination Works

In order to understand how our bodies might shut down the process of urination due to the triggering of the sympathetic system, it is important to understand how the process of urination works normally.

The bladder consists of the *detrusor, urethra, internal sphincter,* and *external sphincter*. The bladder, or detrusor, is the muscular organ that stores urine. It expands as urine collects and contracts as urine expels. The urethra is the muscular canal through which urine passes from the bladder to the outside of the body. Two sphincters also control urination, and both must relax for urine to leave the bladder. The internal sphincter, which is under involuntary control, is located in the neck of the bladder. The external sphincter, which is under voluntary control, is joined to the *pubococcygeal*, or pelvic floor, muscles. Contracting the external sphincter by squeezing the pelvic floor muscles stops urine that has already passed through the internal sphincter, while relaxing the same muscles allows urine to flow.

Urination essentially involves two simultaneous and coordinated processes. For urination to occur, the detrusor muscle of the

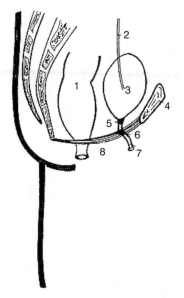

1. Rectum
2. Ureter
3. Bladder
4. Pubic bone
5. Internal Urethral Sphincter
6. External Urethral Sphincter
7. Urethra
8. Pubococcygeus Muscles

Figure 2.2   Lateral view of the urinary system

bladder must contract to expel the urine at the same time that both sphincters relax to release the urine. Both of these processes are affected by the sympathetic nervous system (the involuntary "fight or flight" system). Thus, urination is involuntarily unresponsive under conditions where the sympathetic system is triggered, or aroused. Such arousal in response to a perceived threat produces two physical reactions which prevent urination: relaxation of the detrusor muscle of the bladder, essentially storing the urine instead of expelling it, and contraction of both the internal and external sphincters, which prevents the flow of urine from leaving the bladder. During arousal of the sympathetic system, even if an individual could manually push down on the detrusor and relax the external (voluntary) sphincter, the internal (involuntary) sphincter typically remains contracted, preventing urinary function, until the arousal subsides.

The fact that BBS is psychologically caused is actually good news. Why? Because it means that it is possible to treat BBS with straightforward counseling methods instead of invasive surgical procedures. Many people also find peace of mind when they discover that their BBS is psychological rather than physical:

> *When I first started having problems peeing in bathrooms away from home, I got really worried. I mean, I didn't know what was happening, so I thought I had a bladder tumor or something. Nor had I ever heard anybody talk about this particular problem. . . . Well, I finally went to a urologist and after some interviewing and a series of tests he told me that nothing was physically wrong with me. And did I feel relieved! He then suggested I see a psychologist, and that's when I figured out what was really going on.*

Summary

To summarize the interrelationship of the bladder and brain, the sympathetic system of the autonomic nervous system will physiologically respond to the subconscious perception of a threat in our environment. For those with BBS, the perceived "threat" is most often found in the environment of a rest room while others are nearby. An involuntary physiological response occurs, which prevents the flow of urine by relaxing the detrusor muscle of the bladder and contracting the external and internal sphincters. If you are paruretic, conscious efforts to "will" yourself to override this subconscious, physiological reaction will generally fail as long as your brain perceives the threat in your environment. When you remove yourself from the threatening environment, this "fight or flight" hyper-alert response stops, and urination becomes possible.

CHAPTER THREE

Causes of Bashful Bladder Syndrome: Unraveling the Mystery

If you have bashful bladder syndrome, you may wonder, "Why do I have this?" or "How did this thing get started in the first place?" Unfortunately, there is no consensus concerning the exact causes (or etiology) of BBS among the general public. There appear to be many causes for the onset of BBS, though symptoms can arise following a single event. Another variable is the personal space and comfort threshold every individual possesses:

> I also suffer from this condition and have absolutely no idea why. I think it became more pronounced when I was about fifteen years old. . . . I was recently talking to a friend (who doesn't suffer) and he told me that he was recently subjected to a drug test where an observer was present. He had great difficulty in producing a sample for the test. Could this mean that many, many people suffer and just experience it in certain degrees?

In chapter 1, we hypothesized that when a traumatic incident happens to someone in early adolescence, a pattern of behavior is put into motion. Most paruretics explain their experience in terms of their "plumbing not working," no matter how much they need or want to go, so it is clear that people with paruresis have no voluntary control over being able to urinate in public. The question to be answered, then, is *why* does this involuntary reaction occur in so many people?

How could such a basic human physiological function be so complicated?

Perspectives for Explaining BBS

One thing about BBS is certain: A single root cause that adequately and generally explains the nature of BBS continues to elude clinicians and researchers. BBS is a multifaceted problem, which means its causes—and therefore, therapies—will vary from person to person. While one adult might experience BBS in response to childhood trauma to the urinary system, another might respond to body shyness, and still another to a traumatic event in a rest room. In each instance, however, the manifestation of BBS is the same: the inability to urinate in public rest rooms.

Clinical investigators have offered a variety of perspectives on BBS in the hopes of identifying common aspects of the problem, as well as eventually developing a general treatment program. Because no single explanation is universally applicable, the best way to explain BBS in medical/therapeutic terms is with the *biopsychosocial perspective*.

The Biopsychosocial Perspective

Today, most BBS researchers have a multidimensional philosophy about their work, which they have acquired by considering the relationship between the biological, psychological, and social aspects that affect an individual. The combination of the three perspectives, and how they interrelate, is called the *biopsychosocial perspective*. It is a holistic approach that attributes complex occurrences or events to multiple causes. It also takes into consideration all dynamics—physical, mental, and environmental—that operate on us.

An example of applying the biopsychosocial perspective to a BBS sufferer can be illustrated with the case history of "Mike," a former client of one of the coauthors. Mike grew up in a modest family and was raised to believe that "nice" boys do not "pee" in front of others (social). Later in adulthood, when he experienced conflicts and distress over not being able to urinate in public facilities (psychological), he worried about his urinary "performances" (psychological). Consequently, his nervous system became so triggered, or aroused, in public rest rooms that urination was very difficult (biological). Berating himself about not being able to urinate (psychological), he then avoided accepting extended social invitations that might take him away from his "safe" toilet at home (social).

Thus, the interrelationship of Mike's biopsychosocial system served to create and perpetuate BBS. Like three pieces of a puzzle, the biological, psychological, and social components worked together, creating a full picture of BBS in Mike.

Biological Perspective of BBS

The biological perspective is primarily concerned with the effects of biological and physical processes on BBS. The biological perspective includes a subcategory, the *biochemical perspective*. The biochemical perspective embraces the belief that all aspects of human functioning reflect *biological* and *chemical processes*. Physicians sharing this perspective believe BBS is the result of physical disease, structural problems, or chemical imbalances. They treat BBS by attempting to correct or reverse impaired biological processes by urethral surgery, catheterization, and/or medications.

Two diverging theories within the biochemical approach are the *neural* and *genetic perspectives*. According to the neural perspective, BBS is due to nervous system activity, especially the arousal of the sympathetic autonomic system. Although neural processes are fairly well understood, the functioning of the nervous system as a whole in controlling urinary behavior is not.

Proponents of the genetic perspective believe that most aspects of human functioning are genetically determined prior to birth. They believe that since chromosomes contain genes, the blueprint for the structure and functioning of the body, including urination and its related disturbances, is also genetically determined. In other words, certain people may have a genetic predisposition to developing BBS. This view is consistent with the tendency of the disorder to be found in families. While there are many examples of anecdotes supporting the idea, it is as yet unproven.

Psychological Perspective of BBS

Those who favor the psychological perspective of BBS examine how a lifetime of thoughts, attitudes, emotions, behaviors, and experiences affect urinary functioning. This perspective focuses on the attitude toward urination held by people with BBS ("People will think badly of me if they hear me pee"); openness about discussing the problem ("My family will reject me if I tell them"); how urinary problems develop (conditioning); and methods of influencing these areas, usually through psychotherapy. The psychological perspective has several subcategories.

Psychodynamic Perspective

The psychodynamic perspective is based on Freudian theory. It is the view that our unconscious and repressed motivations and desires determine how we interact in the world. This perspective is similar to the traditional psychiatric perspective. A Freudian psychiatrist and a psychodynamic therapist might consider a person with BBS to have deep-seated hostility toward his or her parents. Such desires, unacceptable to the conscious mind, lead to a "symptom" that prevents the direct expression of hostility. Treatment is by psychoanalysis, which is designed to help lift the patient's repression in order to relieve the urinary symptoms. As most paruretics can attest, a treatment approach that is limited to psychoanalysis is largely unsuccessful.

Cognitive Perspective

The cognitive perspective is held by cognitive theorists. Cognitive theorists believe that thought processes significantly affect our daily lives. This view embraces the idea that our perception of events, as opposed to the actual events, is of primary importance. Behaviorists, by contrast, are concerned with learning theory, or how experience changes our behavior.

Cognitive theorists Middlemist, Knowles, and Matter (1976) emphasized the importance of a paruretic's perception when they proposed that the invasion of personal space was a critical factor in inhibiting urination. In their study, they noted that certain cognitive states—tension, anxiety, and embarrassment—inhibited relaxation of the urethral sphincters. They concluded that certain states of mind could lead to urinary hesitancy, increased bladder pressure, and even acute retention.

Along these lines, one person relates:

> *Associations I have with urinating have to do with*
> *masculinity, that being able to pee anywhere and in front of*
> *anyone belongs to a dominant "macho" image I fall short*
> *of. . . . Perhaps I should think of my own territorial issues,*
> *why I'm afraid to "leave my mark," so to speak.*

Behaviorists usually refer to three types of learning: *classical conditioning* (learning by association), *operant conditioning* (learning by reinforcement and punishment), and *observational learning* (learning by observation and imitation). To a behaviorist, the development of BBS can be illustrated by using the example of "Billy":

Billy observes and learns "modest" urinating behaviors, like always using a stall, from his parents (observational learning). As an older child, his peers tease him about his never using urinals. Eventually, urinating at all in the presence of others becomes associated with teasing and anxiety (classical conditioning). Each time Billy avoids using a public rest room, he further reinforces the problem (operant conditioning).

Cognitive-Behavioral Perspective

Many experts believe that the behavioral perspective is incomplete if the role of thinking is ignored. This position has given rise to the cognitive-behavioral perspective, which combines learning *and* cognitive theories.

Beginning in the 1960s, case reports on treating BBS using a cognitive and behavioral methodology began to appear. The typical treatments included working with clients to challenge and change their distorted perceptions (for example, changing thoughts while urinating in public, from "Everyone is wondering why I'm standing here not peeing" to "No one cares if I pee or not"), and systematic desensitization.

Albert Ellis (1962) developed a form of cognitive-behavioral therapy known as rational-emotive therapy, or "RET," to eliminate irrational beliefs. His method is useful for handling issues of everyday living and has been successfully applied to numerous clinical problems, including social phobias (Zgourides and Warren 1990). More research is needed, however, to determine the effectiveness of RET in treating BBS.

Existential-Humanistic Perspective

The existential-humanistic perspective stresses the importance of immediate experience, self-acceptance, and self-fulfillment. Being (a) aware of, and (b) appropriately able to express emotions like anger and hostility are important aspects of this perspective. Theorists who use the existential-humanistic perspective believe that working on self-acceptance may help paruretics overcome the anxiety in a public rest room that interferes with their ability to urinate.

33

Systems Perspective

The systems perspective is concerned with how different social systems interact and influence individuals, couples, and families. Social workers often refer to this as the "person-in-environment" (PIE) perspective. The most common social systems are family, work, school, community, and religious systems. Many people receive conflicting or unhealthy messages about genitals, urination, and sexuality from their parents, teachers, friends, or religious leaders. For some people, these messages set the stage for the development of paruresis. It can be helpful to identify which system may have provided these erroneous or damaging message(s).

Notice the complex level of interacting events and the impact of systems in this story:

> *I've experienced the following regarding paruresis: hesitancy to urinate in my own apartment, even without another present. Total lack of ability to urinate in front of others except, in a few cases, when heavily intoxicated or heavily stimulated by caffeine. . . . I can urinate in natural settings (in the woods off the highway) as long as I'm aware that another human being is nowhere to be found. I love urinating outside in desolate or woody areas, I feel so natural and there is no pressure on you. This could be stored in our genes somewhere, and modern-day indoor settings may not have evolved into our brains as of yet. I was once given a fifty dollar ticket for urinating in the woods. I could not explain to the cop that I couldn't use a public urinal. . . .*
>
> *The problem already existed when I was in first grade. My mother suffers the same problem as I do. I was hit by a car when I was ten years old and I had to supply a sample of urine in the hospital. I could not perform with my mother in the bathroom and she said she would leave the bathroom and make sure no one came in so I would be able to urinate. She knew I had the problem without me even telling her. . . .*
>
> *Back in college, I always had to trek off to a faraway, infrequently used lavatory, usually causing me to show up to class late, just so I could urinate before attending a long class. . . . I had to skip many office jobs where the lavatories were in busy areas of the office. When I go on interviews, I usually check out the lavatory equipment. . . . I would even leave nightclubs and search desolate factory streets/alleys in Manhattan, just so I could urinate with the hope of not getting jumped by someone possibly in the shadows. The*

problem is always in the back of your mind and you must guide your way through life, accommodating many situations so that they fit your paruresis.

In the example above, the paruresis appears to have had a family component, both physically and as a perpetuator of the problem. With no family discussion, the paruresis continued under the conspiratorial silence between two sufferers of BBS (mother and son). Paruresis was a part of his school experience as early as first grade. The traumatic event of being hit by a car, as related by this person also included the additional trauma of not being able to provide a urine sample. Potential work situations first had to meet the criteria of having acceptable bathroom facilities. Social situations were mitigated by the fear/need to find an acceptable place to relieve himself. The end remark summarizes the impact of all of these things—as for most paruretics, this person's entire life revolves around his paruresis.

Environmental Differences—Sons and Daughters

In the United States, how adults in a family system have traditionally interacted with a young son, as opposed to a young daughter, in public rest room situations raises an interesting issue with regard to paruresis. While females have received consistent "training" and opportunity for observational learning of public toilet habits, males have not.

With few exceptions, adults today were raised as young children in either two-parent homes or divorced homes where the mother was head of household. (It traditionally has not been that common for fathers to have custody of their children in divorce situations.) When in public, the young child—male or female—who needed to use the rest room usually did so by accompanying the mother into the ladies' room. Thus, a son was taught, as was a daughter, to use the public toilet in the privacy of a stall, much as they learned to urinate privately at home. Both male and female young children in day care environments urinate in stand-alone bathrooms. Young children in kindergarten, as well as in first grade, frequently have a private bathroom in the classroom.

So, up until approximately the second grade, boys are exposed to private bathroom environments at home and away from home, whether in public or in day care, just as girls are. Even at school, the stalls provide a familiar option for the boy:

> *The only thing I can think of in my childhood that may have contributed to this problem was an incident that occurred in elementary school. I was urinating in a stall [emphasis ours] and a "bully type" grabbed me from behind and shook me. I think that I urinated everywhere, and may have urinated on myself. I am fairly sure that after this incident, I had trouble voiding in a crowded rest room. I have two brothers, and I know that at least one has a mild case of this, although nowhere near the level of my problem.*

As boys grow a bit older, at around the age of seven or eight, they are no longer taken into the ladies' room when in public because they are "too old," and instead are relegated to the men's room. For the first time in public, young boys are confronted with a much less private urinal situation than the familiar ladies' room stall, and without the comfort of being accompanied by their mother. Adult strangers stand at the urinal while the boys urinate.

There is no doubt that this situation could provoke anxiety in a young male child. If accompanied by a male family member or friend, the boy gains a degree of safety and perhaps the added luxury of being "taught" how to use the urinal. But for the child who has never had the opportunity to learn about the public men's room environment, being confronted with the urinal situation alone for the first time could certainly be traumatic, and could potentially set off the development of BBS.

Social Perspective of BBS

In any group of people, within the diversity of the individuals who constitute the group, there is a cohesiveness of certain attitudes, a collective understanding of what is acceptable or not in day-to-day living. Social perspectives are concerned with social and cultural influences and values.

There are several subcategories of social perspectives: the cross-species, cross-cultural, statistical, and religious perspectives.

Cross-Species Perspective

Because humans are members of the animal kingdom, a comparison between humans and animals can provide valuable insights into the nature of human functioning. The cross-species perspective of BBS considers the similarities in, and differences between, human behavior and that of other animals. While most mammals are fairly solitary, urinating in the presence of other mammals is common. Since the act of urinating for wild animals inherently makes the animal vulnerable to attack, mammals learn early on to urinate in front of other animals. They also learn that there are safe and unsafe times and places to urinate.

Mammals who are more social may remove themselves from others in order to urinate privately or in an "acceptable" environment. Domesticated animals are taught to urinate in specific and acceptable environments. Dogs, for example, are "house-trained" to "hold it" inside a house and are taught that the only safe environment to "go" is "outside." The act of house-training is to teach the dog that going *inside* the house is "unsafe"—e.g., unacceptable and one that may subject the dog to punishment—so the dog will hold its urine until it can urinate freely outdoors, where it receives praise for being "good." The dog is conditioned to perceive the home as an unsafe place to urinate and will not go inside the house. Indeed, the act of house-training is the act of imposing the tenets of paruresis on dogs! (Unfortunately for dog owners, dogs do not seem to share the human tendency to have a onetime learning event.)

Cross-Cultural Perspective

A cross-cultural perspective addresses cultural differences and issues. What may be the norm in one culture may be taboo in another. What is acceptable and common practice among people is relative, based on social expectations and standards of behavior indigenous to a particular culture.

With regard to paruresis, standards of body function, body awareness, and privacy issues differ among cultures. For example, Asians have a reputation for being more modest in their urinary habits than Americans. While we do know that paruresis exists worldwide, we do not yet know if the disorder is more prevalent among certain cultural groups; this area could use more study. Research investigating the incidence of paruresis among cultures with differing attitudes toward the body and its function may yield insights into the dynamics of paruresis.

Statistical Perspective

Statisticians are concerned with identifying the characteristics of the largest number of members in a population, or the "average" person's traits. The information derived from statistical research is commonly reported to the public: The average child consumes X tons of dirt in his or her childhood; the average adult will need X hours of sleep to function optimally; and so on. It is information from two empirical studies that provided the figure that BBS is found in approximately 7 percent of the population, with 10 percent of paruretics critically impaired by BBS to the extent that they experience a significant negative impact on their daily living. The information gleaned from statistical research provides invaluable information in identifying genetic and/or environmental factors that contribute to the development of paruresis.

Religious Perspective

This perspective addresses the effects that religious dogma, doctrine, and scriptures have on us. If you were raised in a religious system, the morals and values set forth by organized religion may play a powerful role in your life—whether healthy or harmful. Religious ideas about family structure and expectations influence communication among family members. In terms of BBS, religion can affect our attitudes toward discussion about "private" body functions and our freedom (or lack thereof) to speak about psychological difficulties or inabilities.

Summary

While there are several theories as to the causes of BBS, there does not appear to be one root cause for the condition. It is evident from case histories that a variety of causes can ultimately lead to the inability to urinate in public rest rooms or in the presence of others. In the search for answers, genetic and psychological functioning and propensities need to be considered. The impact of traumatic episodes and environmental factors, including bathroom design, on the creation of paruresis must also be examined. It is only through extensive research that the causes—and from that, more effective treatments—can be identified and quantified. In the meantime, a multidimensional approach to treatment that encompasses some of the most common causes is the most successful option.

CHAPTER FOUR

You *Can* Treat Bashful Bladder Syndrome Yourself

I am a male professional psychologist, but I also have suffered from bashful bladder for thirty years. . . . If you have had bashful bladder for many years, the chances of psychotherapy working any quick miracles are slim. . . . I spent thousands of dollars on therapy with no long-lasting results. Therapy is an art, and few are really good at it. Even fewer therapists have any experience with bashful bladder.

It seems that every damn doctor I've ever told about my problem was "absolutely certain" that he could cure my problem, that he had the magic bullet. Keep in mind, I've been to see three psychiatrists, a psychologist, a general practitioner, a urologist (as you'd expect, this one found nothing wrong), a hypnotherapist (in addition to one of the psychiatrists who tried hypnotherapy), and a wicca (witch, whatever you want to call her). My best results came through accepting that I had to do something to get over the problem when I took a job in outside sales.

What is the alternative? Continuing to secretly suffer, occasionally seeking the help of professionals who generally don't have a clue about the many levels of difficulties this phobia creates? I'm certainly not saying therapy or hypnosis cannot help. It just appears that thus far none of us have been "cured" by such methods.

As these comments suggest, paruretics know that they need help, and indeed, are anxious to find help that works. The biggest problem paruretics encounter is finding treatment that yields results.

With so few knowledgeable therapists available, along with promises of success that never materialize, it is easy to see why paruretics suffer a tremendous level of frustration and despair in the search for a cure. It also is understandable that many paruretics, having tried so many things that don't work, are reluctant to even attempt any further treatment, instead resigning themselves to merely accommodating this traumatic condition.

But if you suffer from paruresis, don't give up. With all due respect to the frustration and doubt you justifiably feel, there *is* treatment that is effective. The purpose of this chapter is to provide you with definitive help that has worked for many other paruretics. You can work on this problem yourself, or with a therapist if you so choose.

Step One: Where to Start

As with any condition that has a physiological component, the first step in treating BBS is to rule out a purely physical reason for the urinary dysfunction. This requires a visit to a medical professional to make sure that there is no physical impediment to your ability to urinate. If you have had such a physical exam in the past and it was determined that physically your urological system was fine, it is important to make another visit to the doctor before starting BBS treatment. Bodies change, problems can arise, and it is vital not to overlook possible physical causes for your inability to urinate.

A general rule of thumb that should help both you and your physician determine if the cause of your inability to urinate is physical as opposed to psychological is this: If, when alone, you are able to initiate urine easily, maintain a steady stream of urine, and get the feeling that your bladder is empty after finishing, then it is unlikely that your problem urinating is physical. An additional aid to making the determination of BBS is to take the BBS self-test found in chapter 1 of this book.

Step Two: Reviewing the History of Your BBS

After visiting a medical professional and ruling out a physiological cause for your BBS, the next step is to review the nature of your bashful bladder problem in detail. It is helpful to keep a separate journal to record your thoughts about BBS as well as responses to the following exercise.

The purpose of the exercise is merely to provide you with insights into the dynamics of your BBS. Set aside private, quiet time and read the following questions. Write down your answers. There are no right or wrong answers, so write the first thought that comes into your mind:

1. How long have you had this problem?

2. If you recall, how old were you the first time you remember having difficulty urinating?

3. What was going on in your life at the time?

4. Where were you when it happened?

5. Who was with you (family, friends, classmates, strangers)?

6. What happened?

7. How did you feel when it happened the first time?

8. Did you tell anyone? Why or why not?

9. If you told someone, what was his or her reaction?

10. Did your problem not being able to urinate continue totally and immediately after the first instance, or did the symptoms gradually get worse over time?

11. If the problem gradually worsened, did a life-changing event (such as family circumstance, college, job change) have an impact on your symptoms?

12. If so, in what way?

13. Do any family members have the problem?

14. If so, is the problem discussed?

15. Has the problem worsened over time?

16. Are you able to initiate urine in public under any conditions?

17. If so, what conditions?

18. What is your biggest concern now when entering a public rest room?

19. Has that concern changed over the years (i.e., has it become greater, lesser, a different concern)?

20. Do you have recurring negative thoughts when entering a public rest room?

21. If so, what are they?

22. What treatments have you tried so far?

23. What has worked?

24. What hasn't worked?

25. What goal do you now have for treating your BBS?

26. How much confidence do you have that the treatment will help you?

27. Why do you think you do or do not have confidence that the treatment will help?

28. What do you think your life would be like without having BBS as a controlling element of your life?

Take time to think about what you wrote down. The answers may yield significant insight into the dynamics of your BBS. If you are approaching treatment with a therapist, you may want to share your responses to these questions.

Step Three: Understanding Graduated Exposure Therapy

The best evaluated treatment for BBS is referred to as *graduated exposure therapy*. Graduated exposure therapy is widely used for overcoming many fears and phobias, including fears of heights, enclosures, small animals, flying, and driving. The theory behind it is that the more often a person confronts a situation that is frightening, the less frightening the situation becomes. This treatment is based on a simple concept: Do what you fear. However, in order to gain the most benefit from doing what you fear, the object or situation you fear must be confronted *gradually*, often, and for prolonged periods of time.

For paruretics, since the avoidance of urinating in public rest rooms is a large part of the phobia, the "do what you fear" concept of graduated exposure therapy involves gradually and repetitively attempting to urinate in the presence of others, in situations ranging from those which are "safe" to more challenging situations. Exposure sessions should last approximately one hour and should be conducted as often as possible. Multiple sessions each week are preferable, but at least one session weekly is a must.

If you are male, conduct all of your urinating exercises while standing up, aiming directly at the water in order to maximize the sound, without excessive background noise. The reason for this is that buffering urinary noises only makes therapy longer and harder because you are trying to hide/disguise your problem rather than facing it fully.

Step Four: Fluid Loading

In order for graduated exposure therapy to be the most helpful, it is important to try to urinate as many times as possible during each practice session. Consequently, a substantial amount of urine is needed. You know what that means! You will need to drink a lot of fluids, to the point that you feel you are going to burst. This process is called "fluid loading."

The idea of fluid loading goes against one of the main coping mechanisms paruretics use, that is, controlling the intake of fluids in order to control the "when and where" of needing to urinate. However, for treatment purposes, the increased urgency will facilitate your ability to urinate, and thus your success in doing so. Fluid loading is a critical step in graduated exposure therapy for BBS and cannot be skipped or minimized.

Keep in mind that everyone differs in the amount of fluid needed to feel urinary urgency. Some people need to drink a lot of fluids; some may not need to drink much at all. The type of fluids you choose to drink is up to you, but many paruretics find that water, tea, and coffee work best. One cautionary note: Do not *overload* on fluids!

Step Five: Keeping an Urgency Scale

In order to keep track of your success with various levels of urgency, you will need to keep an *urgency scale*. After fluid loading, use a scale of zero to ten to rate your physical sense of urinary urgency, with zero indicating no urgency and ten equaling extreme urgency. Do not try your initial exposure exercises until your urgency is at the level of seven or above.

Step Six: The "Buddy"

Secrecy about paruresis is common among most paruretics, and is understandable given the embarrassing nature of the problem. However, in treating BBS it is invaluable to have a partner, or "buddy." The buddy can be a professional therapist or a trusted family member or friend. If you know someone else who has BBS, you can serve as buddies to one another.

The role of the buddy is simple: He or she will stand at various distances from you (whatever your comfort threshold will allow), in various bathroom environments, as you attempt to urinate. You give your buddy directions on where to stand. You are in control of your buddy's movements toward you during the graduated exposure process.

If you do not feel comfortable having a buddy, it is best to begin imagining someone next to you or to choose isolated public rest rooms where a person may occasionally walk past the rest room door.

For purposes of this description of self-treatment, we shall assume you have engaged the assistance of a buddy.

Step Seven: Exposure Process— Beginning BBS Exercise

Through exposure therapy, you will learn to urinate in gradually more challenging locations. The starting point for your exposure therapy is to identify in which situation you are able to successfully urinate. The critical issue is to begin your self-treatment session in a situation where you feel confident that you will be successful.

You may be thinking that there is not *any* situation where you are confident of success. That's okay. If you cannot be confident at all, then determine the *least difficult* situation for *you* and start working on your problem from that point. For example, you might begin at home alone and imagine people are standing next to you while you use the toilet.

A basic concept of graduated exposure therapy is repetition. You should repeat a successful trial *two times* before moving onto a more difficult exercise. At any given point that you are unsuccessful, go back to the last point, where you *were* successful and try again at that point until you are successful two more times.

Many paruretics say that they are able to urinate in an isolated public rest room (a single commode with a locked door). Thus, a single facility rest room is a good starting point for your graduated exposure. Have your buddy stand outside the door at a distance that feels comfortable to you. Enter the rest room, close the door firmly, and attempt to urinate.

If you are successful, allow the urine to flow for approximately three seconds and then *stop* the flow. The reason for this three-second limit is that you will need to save your urine for repeated exposure attempts. Remember, each exposure session will involve several attempts at urinating.

If you are unsuccessful in initiating urine, wait by the toilet for two minutes. If you still are unable to go, take a three-minute break. (However, if at the end of the two minutes, you feel as if you are just about to urinate, wait no longer than two more minutes; after this second attempt, whether successful or not, take a three-minute break.) If you continue to not be able to initiate a urine stream, open the door and direct your buddy to move farther away from the door, close the door firmly, and attempt to urinate. If you find that you are still unable to initiate urine at all during your session, don't worry about it. Simply end the session and try again in a few days. Next time, try either a more isolated location or your home bathroom.

If you are able to urinate with your buddy outside the door one time, take a break of approximately three minutes and repeat the process. Have your buddy stand at the point at which you were successful the first time while you repeat the process. *Remember: Always start at the point where you were successful before moving on to another situation.*

Once you are able to successfully urinate two times with your buddy outside the door, repeat the process having your buddy move closer toward the door, until you are able to successfully urinate two times with your buddy just outside the closed door. *Remember: You are in control of the distance between the two of you.* Because many paruretics have experienced boundary violations at some point or another, which may be in part responsible for their condition, this is a very important rule. *Never* bring your buddy closer than you feel comfortable at that moment.

Step Eight: Advanced Graduated Exposure Exercises

Once you have has mastered the ability to urinate with your buddy just outside the closed door, the next step is to open the rest room door slightly. At this point, tell your pee buddy to move a distance away from the door. Once you have successfully urinated two times with the door slightly ajar, direct your pee buddy to stay in the same position and open the door a little more. Repeat this exercise, gradually opening the door a little each time, until you are able to urinate with your pee buddy at a distance and the door fully open. Remember, after each trial you should take a break, whether you were able to initiate a urine stream or not.

After you have mastered the ability to urinate with the door fully open and your buddy at a distance, the next exercise is to allow your partner to gradually approach the door. A few feet at a time is best. Do not allow your partner to move closer until you have succeeded at least twice in a row at a given distance. Continue allowing your buddy to approach you until he or she is standing directly behind you as you attempt to urinate.

Once you are able to successfully urinate two times with your partner standing directly behind you, have your partner make noise or impatient comments while you attempt to urinate. This experience will help prepare you for any rude behavior you may encounter in a public rest room.

The next step after mastering urinating in a private setting with your partner behind you is to visit isolated public rest rooms with your partner. If you are a man, you should practice at the urinal; there is no need to repeat the exercises in the stall.

Step Nine: You're on Your Own

After several successful trials in isolated public rest rooms with your buddy present, you are ready to complete the treatment on your own. If you haven't used a partner up until this point, the treatment from here forward is the same as for those who did decide to engage the assistance of a partner.

It is at this point in self-treatment that something amusing may happen. Instead of waiting for people to *leave* the rest room, the paruretic ironically has to wait for people to *come into* the rest room, to serve as opportunities to practice urinating. The best strategy at this point is to wait discreetly outside a public rest room that has a light to moderate flow of people. Once someone enters the rest room, enter the rest room yourself and attempt to urinate before the other person leaves. If the other person leaves before you can get started, simply step out of the rest room and wait for another opportunity.

After you have succeeded several times with others present in stalls and at the other urinals, the next step is to attempt to urinate in a more crowded rest room. Try urinating at the mall, a busy airport, a sporting event, a concert, the theater, or a building on campus. Once you are able to master these crowded situations, the last phase of treatment is the *maintenance phase*.

Step Ten: Maintenance Phase

The maintenance phase of treatment involves continuing to practice in public rest rooms with other people present. We recommend urinating in one public rest room daily for at least thirty days after completing the formal exposure sessions. Once the thirty-day period of daily attempts is over, it is prudent to take advantage of any opportunity to urinate with people nearby whenever possible.

Frequently Asked Questions about Graduated Exposure Therapy for BBS

How many sessions are usually required to get me to the point where I'm practicing in crowded rest rooms?

In our clinical experience, with trained therapeutic assistance, the average number of sessions required is between eight and twelve. Remember that *these are just average figures*. Some of our patients make progress with fewer sessions; others require substantially more. The important issue is not how many sessions it takes, but what pace is comfortable for *you*. Be persistent, and your chances of improvement are great.

This sounds too simple and too good to be true. How can this work?

Graduated exposure therapy for BBS works by retraining the brain to realize that urinating in front of others is not threatening. Think about it. At some point in time, you were able to urinate in public. Through triggering event(s), your brain learned to not allow you to urinate in public. This process provides your brain with information that it is okay to urinate in what used to be perceived as a threatening environment.

What do I do if I'm unable to urinate after several attempts at a particular step in the exposure process?

First of all, relax. You're not alone. Most people with BBS do *not* progress smoothly from one step to the next in relearning to urinate with others present. That is why the treatment includes not moving on until you have successfully repeated an exercise two times. If, however, you seem "stuck" at a particular level of exposure, it is best to persist with a given step several times before trying something easier. Retreating quickly can lead to backsliding and staying stuck at a particular level of exposure, so try to avoid retreating once treatment is fully underway. *This advice does NOT apply when you are just starting out and are trying to find your initial treatment starting point.*

What do I do if my treatment progress stalls for a prolonged period of time and I cannot go in any given trial situation?

If you find that you are stalled for a prolonged period of time, there are two options. One is to continue to attempt this step, session after session, until you achieve your goal. If, after repeated persistence, you are still stalled in your progress, the other option is to add other treatments. These treatments might include counseling designed to change your thinking, known as *cognitive restructuring*, and/or using relaxation techniques (discussed in more detail in chapter 5). In addition, if progress in therapy comes to a halt, a second medical evaluation should be considered to be certain there is not an underlying medical cause.

What happens if I have loaded up on fluids for a session and cannot urinate the entire time?

If this happens to you, do not panic. Remove yourself from the trial session environment and go to a location that is less challenging. This may mean using your bathroom at home, a location that is generally "safe" for paruretics.

In extremely rare instances (we know of only one such case), paruretics may not be able to relieve themselves during or after a self-conducted exposure session. If this happens, go to a hospital emergency room and have a catheter used to relieve your bladder.

How effective is graduated exposure therapy for BBS?

Graduated exposure therapy for BBS was designed and developed at the University of Michigan Anxiety Disorders Program. At this program, approximately 75 percent of BBS patients obtained substantial improvement in their ability to urinate in public rest rooms.

Of the last twenty-six BBS patients who were treated with graduated exposure therapy, twelve males were able to consistently urinate at the urinal with others behind or beside them, eight males were able to urinate at the urinal with others behind or beside them most of the time, four were able to urinate with others behind or beside them occasionally, and two did not improve at all. The average number of sessions completed was just over nine, although one patient required thirty-three sessions to obtain the ability to urinate with others behind or beside him.

When the patients were contacted several months after ending treatment, approximately 40 percent had further improvement, 40 percent had regressed somewhat, although rarely back to pre-treatment functioning, and approximately 20 percent maintained the same level of improvement that was achieved at the end of treatment.

Most of the paruretics in this group were treated with one session weekly. Seven of the groups were treated with nine exposure sessions completed over a five-day period because these individuals attended the clinic from out of town, necessitating a one-week concentrated program. The paruretics from out of town achieved a similar rate of improvement when compared to those who received single weekly sessions.

Moreover, the International Paruresis Association has sponsored a number of weekend workshops based on the graduated exposure methods developed at the University of Michigan. The results of these workshops are very encouraging as well. Results from the twenty-seven participants so far include:

- Prior to the workshop, on a zero to ten scale (one the least, ten the most), participants averaged 6.75 in their own assessment of the severity of their paruresis. After the workshop, this average decreased to 5.7, and six months later, it was about the same, indicating that the gains held.

- Based on post workshop survey results, *everyone* experienced some improvement, 20 percent felt it helped them some, 50 percent felt it helped a lot, and 30 percent felt it helped enormously.

- Six months later, 5 percent felt it helped a little, 20 percent felt it helped some, 45 percent felt it helped a lot, and 30 percent felt it helped enormously, indicating a slight erosion in gains from the workshop.

These results indicate that the weekend workshop format is a highly effective format for treating paruretics. Key reasons for this are the safety created, the trust that is built up between participants, and the heavy emphasis on practice sessions (seven to eight throughout the weekend). The key long-term change that comes about at the workshop for most people is a cognitive shift, brought about by the behavioral work, that the person is okay if he or she can't urinate in a certain situation, and that it is *not* the end of the world if they aren't successful in certain situations.

Case History: Mr. C—Using Graded Exposure Therapy

Mr. C, a former client of one of the coauthors, is a forty-three-year-old divorced male who is an owner of a very successful fencing company. He lives with his girlfriend. He reports having had difficulty urinating at a urinal with others beside him as far back as he can remember. His problem worsened at the age of forty. He believes that the increased difficulty is related to excessive work stress and a back injury incurred while skiing.

When Mr. C first arrived at the clinic, he could not urinate under any circumstances in public rest rooms unless no one was present and the chances of someone entering seemed remote. He reported that he avoided many situations, including travel away from home, concerts, movies, sporting events, and dates with women that lasted for more than a few hours. He also reported problems at work, since meeting with potential customers often required trips to unfamiliar places at some distances from the office. Mr. C had a private rest room with extra soundproofing built just outside of his office, which made it possible for him to urinate while at work.

Mr. C reported a good childhood. He had many friends and was successful in sports and with his grades. He played baseball in college. Apart from his bashful bladder difficulties, he had no other significant fears that interfered with his life. He did report a fifteen-year history of generalized anxiety for which he was taking tranquilizing medications as needed. The tranquilizers did not help him urinate more easily in public rest rooms.

After completing a full psychiatric evaluation, Mr. C was asked to return for his first session one week later. He was instructed to drink one quart of water one hour prior to the session to induce urinary urgency. When Mr. C arrived at the clinic he rated his urgency an eleven on an urgency scale of zero to ten. Mr. C used a professional therapist as his exposure partner.

The exposure therapy began with the therapist waiting in the hallway approximately ten feet from the door of a private rest room that Mr. C occupied, the door firmly closed. Mr. C was unable to initiate urine within the two-minute waiting time for the first three attempts. By the end of the session, he was able to initiate a halting stream of urine while the therapist remained in the hallway, away from the door.

At the conclusion of the second session, Mr. C was able to initiate a strong stream of urine with the therapist just outside the closed rest room door. By the end of session four, Mr. C was able to initiate urine with the therapist approximately ten feet from the rest room door, with the door opened a slight crack.

During session five, Mr. C was unable to initiate urine under any circumstances, regardless of the fact that his urgency was strong. He reported being under stress the past week.

By session seven, Mr. C was able to urinate with the therapist standing directly behind him. Mr. C canceled session eight because he did not feel strong urgency to urinate. Session nine concluded with Mr. C being able to successfully initiate urine several times while the therapist was directly behind him making noise and anxiety-provoking comments. At this point, Mr. C said that for the first time in his life there seemed to be a "connection" between his bladder and his brain.

Sessions ten through thirteen were spent attempting to urinate in other locations around the medical center, beginning in isolated rest rooms and ending at a crowded rest room near the cafeteria during the noon rush. Sessions fourteen and fifteen were conducted at the university student union during the noon rush of students. The student union rest rooms were especially challenging since there were no partitions between the urinals. The exposure sessions in the medical center and the student union included only a few unsuccessful attempts and all sessions ended only after a successful attempt.

At the end of session fifteen, Mr. C received homework assignments. The homework included two exposure trips to the nearby international airport and daily visits to restaurants and malls in the area. Mr. C was able to complete the assignments within one week and reported near flawless performance.

Mr. C then received his maintenance homework: to enter one public rest room daily after drinking water and obtaining at least a moderate urgency. At follow-up, Mr. C reported that he "had his life back," followed by the correction that he "had his life for the first time."

Summary

Graduated exposure therapy is a valuable therapeutic tool that paruretics can use to overcome the symptoms of BBS. It is a tool that can be used in conjunction with other forms of therapy. Graduated exposure can be done individually, in a group, and/or with a pee buddy. The self-treatment is individualized and progresses according to the paruretic's successes at graduated levels of exposure. Graduated exposure therapy has been shown to be successful in approximately 75–80 percent of cases involving BBS.

CHAPTER FIVE

Adjunct Therapies, Support Groups, and Workshops

In addition to graduated exposure therapy, supportive therapies and peer assistance can be helpful. If you suffer from BBS, cognitive restructuring therapy, relaxation techniques, support groups, and twelve-step programs are resources that can aid you immensely in your search for management and eradication of your symptoms.

Cognitive Restructuring Therapy

Cognitive restructuring therapy is primarily concerned with what a person is thinking when feeling anxious. The therapy involves identifying distorted, inaccurate thoughts and replacing them with more truthful self-statements. This therapy is useful for paruretics, because paruretics frequently experience inaccurate and unrealistic thinking when confronted with the possibility of urinating in a public rest room. "Everyone is watching me here at the urinal," "It will be awful if I can't go," "I just know that I will fail," "I'm such a weak person," and "Everyone thinks I'm strange because I can't urinate" are common thoughts. Most people with BBS accept these statements on faith, without ever having investigated whether or not they are true.

The first step in cognitive therapy for BBS is identifying what thoughts are going through your head when you are attempting to urinate or even when you just think about using a public rest room. You can identify your distorted thoughts by visiting a public rest room and then paying attention to your thinking, or by trying to remember what thoughts were present during a recent situation that was particularly difficult for you. (You may want to refer to your responses to questions 20 and 21 in your BBS history, found in chapter 4.) If you are having trouble identifying your thoughts, consider seeking help from a trained cognitive therapist, or someone who specializes in helping others change distorted thinking.

Once an inaccurate thought is identified, such as "It'll be a catastrophe if I can't go," your job is to find evidence *against* the thought. You can then use the evidence to counter the inaccurate thought that occurs when you enter a challenging rest room situation. In other words, you are to consciously attack the appearance of a negative thought that your subconscious presents to you as you visit a public rest room with evidence that dispels the negative thought.

One source of evidence that can be used to dispel distorted thinking is your own experience. For example, if you think "It'll be a catastrophe if I can't go," realize that while having rest room failures is admittedly disturbing, such failures do not reach the level of "catastrophe." If one of your distorted thoughts is "Everyone is watching me having difficulty urinating," attempt to identify an instance where someone actually did notice that you could not urinate and then criticized you. Most paruretics cannot produce evidence that anyone even *noticed* they could not urinate, let alone that anyone who may have noticed even cared. In the rare event that a person *did* notice and *did* say something, remind yourself that such a remark is a reflection on the other person's rudeness, not your problem.

Another source of information that is extremely helpful in countering your inaccurate thinking is the experience of other paruretics. In treating over 100 patients with paruresis, we found that "terrible" consequences associated with not being able to urinate in front of others are exceedingly rare. The worst-case scenario, if someone says something embarrassing to you, is it is merely that—embarrassing. It is not a catastrophe. Your world will not end. The embarrassing situation, however, will.

A third source of information that is helpful is the use of a *behavioral experiment*. A behavioral experiment is a controlled decision to create a certain behavior and then to observe the reaction to that behavior. For male paruretics, one behavioral experiment would be to enter a rest room and deliberately stand at the urinal *without* urinating. Observe others around you to see if they notice, and if they do, whether they seem to care. With enough practice standing at the urinal for extended periods of time without urinating, you will discover that others really do not pay much attention. Most people have other things to worry about—including going themselves! As part of one man's behavioral experiment, he found it very helpful to say out loud that he was having problems urinating. Contrary to what he expected to hear in response, many people in the rest room said that they have had the problem on occasion as well!

Another behavioral experiment involves the use of the buddy. As your buddy stands near you while you attempt to urinate, observe other people's reaction to your buddy deliberately not urinating. This will give you a chance to see that others do not seem to pay much attention, if any.

These experiences will help you on other occasions when you find yourself becoming excessively concerned about whether people are noticing your urinary difficulties.

For people with bashful bladder problems who experience distorted thoughts that extend beyond the bathroom situation and include such inaccurate thoughts as "I'm a weak person," "I'm a freak," "Someone will think I'm gay if I take too long," or "My life is completely screwed up because I have this problem," the same cognitive restructuring therapy can be used. Rebuke the negative, distorted thoughts with evidence that gives you some perspective.

If the negative thoughts are too strong to overcome on your own, seek professional help from a trained cognitive therapist.

While cognitive restructuring techniques have not been evaluated or proven as a *primary* treatment for paruresis, it is a helpful addition to graduated exposure therapy, especially if you have not responded successfully to graduated exposure therapy alone.

Applied Relaxation Therapy

Applied relaxation therapy is a method devised by Ost (1987). It is a systematic and gradual method of learning how to relax. The applied relaxation procedure has several steps. It is important to note that, as with cognitive restructuring therapy, applied relaxation therapy has been demonstrated to be helpful for many anxiety conditions, but it has never been formally tested as a treatment for paruresis. However, clinical work suggests that a modified version of applied relaxation may be a good supplemental therapy to graduated exposure therapy, when the latter alone has not worked. These techniques should also prove beneficial for those who have difficulty defecating in public rest rooms.

Step One: Awareness of Anxiety

The first step in applied relaxation therapy is to become sensitive to early signs of anxiety. As a paruretic, you should watch for early signs of anxiety associated with urinating. This awareness then serves as a cue to begin relaxing. It is helpful to keep a written record of feelings of anxiety related to urinating. For instance, you may note that you felt anxious when your bladder was very full and you were far away from home.

Step Two: Muscle Tension and Relaxation

The second step in applied relaxation therapy is a physical relaxation technique. By alternately tensing and relaxing a muscle group, you should learn how to consciously distinguish the difference between a state of relaxation versus muscle tension. The exercise is as follows:

1. Lie down and close your eyes.

2. Concentrate on your hands. Tense your hands for five to ten seconds and then relax them for five to ten seconds.

3. Concentrate on the muscles in your forearms. Tense these muscles for five to ten seconds and then relax them for five to ten seconds.

4. Concentrate on your upper arm muscles. Tense these muscles for five to ten seconds and then relax them for five to ten seconds.

5. Repeat the deliberate tensing and relaxing of muscles for 5 to 10 seconds in your forehead, squinting your eyes, crinkling your nose, and clenching your jaw.

6. Repeat the deliberate tensing and relaxing of muscles for five to ten seconds in your neck, shoulders, stomach, lower back, buttocks, upper legs, lower legs, and finally your feet.

It is important to produce tension that is noticeable, but not to the degree that there is pain or injury. If tensing a muscle group produces any pain, skip it and move on to the next group of muscles.

This exercise usually takes about twenty minutes to complete. Some people report that it is helpful to play tapes of nature sounds, such as waterfalls or ocean waves, while practicing this technique. You should do this exercise on a daily basis for two weeks.

Step Three: Release-Only Phase

The next step is a shorter version of the previous exercise: the release-only phase. The goal in Step Three is to further decrease the amount of time it takes to relax by discontinuing the tension portion of the exercise. Instead of tensing first and relaxing afterward, concentrate on relaxing the muscle groups one at a time. This phase should take about seven to ten minutes to complete. If you are having difficulty relaxing a particular muscle group, apply tension as you did in step two until you are able to relax. It is best to practice this step in the therapy daily for two weeks.

Step Four: Cue-Controlled/Conditioned Relaxation

Cue-controlled relaxation, or conditioned relaxation, is the next step. The goal here is to further reduce the time it takes to achieve a state of relaxation. This stage focuses on learning to relax using the self-instruction, "relax." It is accomplished by doing the following:

1. Begin each practice session by first using the release-only technique until you feel relaxed.

2. Focus on your breathing. Take in deep breaths and, just as you are about to release the air, say the word "relax" to yourself as you let the tension leave your body.

3. With each breath, try to imagine tension being gradually released from your body.

4. If you notice that a particular muscle group is tense, focus on it and try to gradually release the tension from that area.

You should practice cue-controlled relaxation several times daily for two weeks.

Step Five: Rapid Relaxation

In this next step of treatment, called *rapid relaxation*, use the anxiety-triggering thoughts you identified previously as a signal to invoke a brief relaxation state. When you notice your anxiety increasing, take one to three deep breaths, and then think the word "relax" before exhaling. Do this while mentally scanning the body for tension and trying to relax as much as possible.

Step Six: Application Training

The final phase in the applied relaxation technique is referred to as *application training*. This phase takes the relaxation skills you have been practicing and applies those skills in rest room situations. From the time that you begin to approach the rest room to the end of your practice attempt, use the rapid relaxation technique to keep your anxiety under control. The goal is to use the relaxation techniques at the first sign of being upset. Scan your body for tension and use the tension as a signal to begin the rapid relaxation procedure described in Step Five. Focus your concentration on releasing the tension your body scan identified. If you have difficulty releasing the tension, use the deliberate tension and relaxation method described in Step Two.

Two Brief Relaxation Exercises

Some people may find it helpful to practice relaxation techniques in order to reduce their anxiety levels before heading into a bathroom. Just paying attention to and labeling your anxiety as unrealistic, and then *deeply breathing through it*, may help your body relax enough to be able to urinate.

Before going into a public rest room, taking time to relax and get yourself centered can be of enormous value. Here are two favorite, quick (about ten minutes) relaxation procedures. The first is found in Johnson (1997):

Get comfortable.

You are going to count backwards from ten to zero.
Silently say each number as you exhale.
As you count, you will relax more deeply and go deeper
     and deeper into a state of relaxation.
When you reach zero, you will be completely relaxed.

You feel more and more relaxed, you can feel the tension
     leave your body.
You are becoming as limp as a rag doll, the tension is
     going away.
You are very relaxed.

Now drift deeper with each breath, deeper and deeper.
Feel the deep relaxation all over and continue relaxing.
Now, relaxing deeper you should feel an emotional calm.

Tranquil and serene feelings, feelings of safety and
security, and a calm peace.

Try to get a quiet inner confidence.
A good feeling about yourself and relaxation.
Study once more the feelings that come with relaxation.
Let your muscles switch off, feel good about everything.
Calm and serene surroundings make you feel more and
more tranquil and peaceful.
You will continue to relax for several minutes.
When I tell you to start, count from one to three, silently
say each number as you take a deep breath.
Open your eyes when you get to three. You will be relaxed
and alert.
When you open your eyes you will find yourself back in
the place where you started your relaxation.
The environment will seem slower and more calm.
You will be more relaxed and peaceful.
Now count from one to three.

The following "deep breathing" exercise can be found in Davis,
Eshelman, and McKay (1995):

1. Although this exercise can be practiced in a variety of
   poses, the following is recommended: Lie down on a
   blanket or rug on the floor. Bend your knees and move
   your feet about eight inches apart with your toes turned
   slightly outward. Make sure that your spine is straight.

2. Scan your body for tension.

3. Place one hand on your abdomen and one hand on
   your chest.

4. Inhale slowly and deeply through your nose into your
   abdomen to push up your hand as much as feels comfortable. Your chest should move only a little and only
   with your abdomen.

5. When you feel at ease with step 4, smile slightly and
   inhale through your nose and exhale through your
   mouth, making a quiet, relaxing, whooshing sound like
   the wind as you blow gently out. Your mouth, tongue,
   and jaw will be relaxed. Take long, slow, deep breaths
   that raise and lower your abdomen. Focus on the sound
   and feeling of breathing as you become more and more
   relaxed.

6. Continue deep breathing for about five or ten minutes at a time, once or twice a day, for a couple of weeks. Then, if you like, extend this period to twenty minutes.

7. At the end of each deep breathing session, take a little time to once more scan your body for tension. Compare the tension you feel at the conclusion of the exercise with that which you experienced when you began.

8. When you become at ease with breathing into your abdomen, practice it at any time during the day when you feel like it and you are sitting down or standing still. Concentrate on your abdomen moving up and down, the air moving in and out of your lungs, and the feeling of relaxation that deep breathing gives you.

9. When you have learned to relax yourself using deep breathing, practice it whenever you feel yourself getting tense.

Distraction Techniques

Some paruretics report that they find various methods of distracting themselves to be valuable when trying to use public rest rooms. Distraction techniques include such actions as counting, holding your breath, looking at a watch, and listening to the tap water run.

Relying on this technique can be negative in the long run, even if it produces short-term results. If you are in a high anxiety-producing situation, then this technique may be useless. It is also commonly reported that distraction techniques cease being effective rather quickly.

More significantly, this technique can interfere with graduated exposure therapy. There is substantial evidence that it can actually hinder that therapy's progress. Given that graduated exposure therapy is the best treatment for BBS currently available, we advise against distraction techniques.

Urinary Self-Catheterization

A viable solution to managing BBS is urinary self-catheterization. Self-catheterization was first used by urologists to teach individuals with spinal cord injuries who could not urinate on their own to use "clean, intermittent self-catheterization" to relieve themselves.

The self-catheterization technique was first recommended for paruretics by coauthor George Zgourides (1996). If you are physically and psychologically able to use self-catheterization, it is an absolute, sure fire method of emptying the bladder. Clients report that it sounds much worse and more painful than it really is, especially in contrast to the alternative of prolonged bladder pain.

Some mental health professionals believe that catheters can be a critical component when used in conjunction with graduated exposure therapy. By learning to self-cath before attempting graduated exposure therapy, they believe that the paruretic always has a safe "out." There is no risk of a trip to the emergency room, and the anxiety level is reduced, helping the effectiveness of the exposure. Men using self-caths while standing at a urinal simulate urinating at a urinal. The experience teaches you that no one pays attention or cares, and that no catastrophe happens, thus relieving two major concerns.

If you are interested in learning more about this method of managing BBS, you need to see your medical provider. A physician or nurse practitioner can easily and quickly teach you the procedure and can prescribe numbing ointments to desensitize the urethra. While catheters are widely available without a prescription, they should *never* be used without first discussing the option with a medical provider and obtaining professional instruction.

This method is *not* for everyone, especially those with structural injuries or who are prone to bladder infections. And while some professionals see self-catheterization as helping graduated exposure therapy, it is by no means a requirement of that therapy. But for those paruretics who take comfort in taking a catheter pack with them on travels away from home, it may provide peace of mind, whether they use it or not.

Yankee Ingenuity

As successful as graduated exposure therapy is, there are times it does not work. When nothing works—including counseling, graduated exposure and relaxation therapies, drugs, biofeedback, psychoanalysis—creativity and Yankee ingenuity come into play. By examining the lifestyle needs of the paruretic who does not respond to known treatments, sometimes the best answer is the most accommodating one.

For example, Zgourides once had a client (we'll call him "John") who had no success whatsoever, no matter which treatment he tried. In reviewing John's lifestyle and biggest problem with BBS, it seemed that his worst complaint was not being able to urinate on long road trips associated with his work. John would sometimes have to drive ten to twelve hours without being able to relieve himself.

After doing a little research, Dr. Zgourides and John came up with the idea of buying a sleeping camper to attach to John's truck. John found an inexpensive camper that allowed him to go inside, close and lock the door, and use his own personal traveling bathroom. Today, John travels all over the country, drinking coffee and sodas without worry and stopping at roadside parks whenever he needs to use his camper toilet.

Follow-up Therapy

After choosing a method of therapy to manage BBS, paruretics as a group typically benefit from continuing to talk about their successes and failures in dealing with the problem. Follow-up therapy fills the need for this type of support. Since BBS is a stubborn problem, gains that are made can disappear without appropriate maintenance therapies. Some paruretics attend therapy as infrequently as a few times a year, while others contact their therapists whenever they have a relapse. As with any other therapy-based treatment, clients and therapists need to outline a relapse prevention program including ongoing and situational support.

Support Groups

Support groups can be invaluable sources of comfort and assurance for paruretics. Since a major component of BBS is secrecy, the relief that can be gained from finally sharing BBS experiences with others who understand and, more to the point, *know firsthand what it is to live with BBS*, can be an overwhelming aid in working toward beating this phobia. The collective experiences of the support group foster a greater understanding of BBS. The perspective gained from listening to others' stories of suffering from BBS reinforces the understanding that you are *not* the only one who has this, you are not crazy, weak, or weird, or less of a person because you cannot urinate publicly. Sharing information about what works and what doesn't can yield treatment or accommodation insights that may work for you, too.

Hooking up with pee buddies who are also paruretic is a great way to institute the self-treatment techniques described in chapter 4.

At this time, there are not many support groups for paruretics. We know of support groups in: Baltimore, Boston, Chicago, Los Angeles, New Jersey/New York, Philadelphia, Portland (Oregon), Seattle, and London (United Kingdom). More are springing up every month. The International Paruresis Association keeps a running list of support groups. The IPA is also in the process of publishing a "how-to" manual for setting up a paruresis support group.

The initiative to create a support group is a difficult first step. Yet, by reaching out to other people who suffer from paruresis, the problem is ultimately lessened for everyone. One client advocated approaching a support group with a "twelve-step" program based on the AA model:

> *I've realized that I'm not sure if I can continue to live this way. Perhaps that's something most of us (especially people trying to cope with extreme cases) need to think about. The thought of giving up so much in life because of this phobia makes me wonder if I'm truly living. I've had relationships strained, passed on job opportunities, missed concerts and sporting events, given up hunting and other activities where I might have to go in front of people, etc. This phobia has in many ways controlled me. It has defined who I am to a large degree. Again, this is something I feel that we need to admit. From these and other realizations, I've concluded that what would be most helpful is a support group similar to twelve-step programs. Obviously, the first step of AA would apply to us, with a minor modification: "Admit that we're powerless over paruresis, that our lives have become unmanageable." This is a very serious "disease." As serious as alcoholism. I've dealt with alcoholism and mental illness in relatives, two painful relationships ending, a spell of unemployment, and countless other difficulties. None compare to the pain and fear of dealing with this secret. Like AA and Alanon, and countless other twelve-step groups, the first step would be to admit powerlessness. Later on, as trust and fellowship develops, we could move on to the next phase, helping each other to work through this phobia.*

Support groups work. Letting go of the stranglehold of secrecy that BBS demands is an important step in gaining back control over your life and defeating this phobia.

Starting a Support Group

There are many books that have been written on the topic of self-help support groups. Two of our favorites are Silverman (1980) and Kurtz (1997). Our goal here is to give you the basics of how to get one started. If you need more help, please contact the International Paruresis Association, listed in resource appendix C.

One of the best ways to start is to simply find a buddy (preferably someone with the same problem, in this case) to form a two-person support group. You can easily practice most of the advice and techniques suggested in this book with the other person. Of course, this will be much easier to do with a same gender partner.

Once you have someone else working with you on a regular basis, you can begin to figure out how to add more people to your group. Once you're up to three, you're a bona fide support group. Since not everyone can make every meeting, you probably want to have a core group of at least six. A group of seven or more *regular* attendees will probably get unwieldy.

Each support group needs a leader or coordinator. Although it would be ideal if everyone took equal responsibility for these functions, for example calling and/or e-mailing reminders about meetings, coordinating dates, and dealing with issues that arise, in reality this rarely happens. So, if you are interested in seeing a group get started, you become the leader! You make it happen.

In our experience, the best model is for a support group to meet regularly, at the same time and day of the week or month if possible. Some groups meet weekly, other bi-monthly, or monthly. In between meetings, group members can pair up for buddy sessions, too.

Once your group is established and meeting at a regular time, you can think of expanding it. The best source of referrals will be other paruretics whom group members know. After this, you can try placing a free public service announcement in your local newspaper and on the radio; FM stations that cater to the twenty-to-fifty crowd work best.

The hardest part in setting up any support group is to get firm commitments from people that they will show up each time (barring emergencies). It can be harmful to the group, affecting morale, if people drift in and out, unless you have a large list of contacts (usually fifteen or more) and can expect four to seven people to show up at any meeting.

People do not like to commit to things, especially something that is going to challenge them and possibly make them anxious or fearful. Plus, paruretics have engaged in avoidance behavior for years, and this is one more thing that they might want to especially avoid!

What should happen at a support group meeting? Someone, usually the person organizing the meeting, should host the meeting at their house. The very first meeting should devote a lot of time to people sharing stories. Then, someone who is versed in graduated exposure methods should *demonstrate* for group members how people should practice these desensitization techniques. It is *not* recommended for people to actually practice during this first session.

At subsequent meetings, the pattern should be for people to review how things are going concerning their paruresis, and then devote the rest of the time for everyone to practice graduated exposure techniques. We cannot emphasize enough that the purpose of support group meetings is to *practice*, not to chitchat. At least two to three hours should be set aside, depending on the size of the group, so that everyone can practice the techniques outlined in this book a number of times (ideally, one to fifteen practices for each person).

At first, meetings should be held at someone's home which has enough bathrooms to accommodate the number of people in the group. For every three people, there should be one bathroom. People should rotate so that everyone gets comfortable urinating behind them. Then, *and only then*, should groups of three venture out together to semi-public and public bathrooms of increasing difficulty. This may mean that one support group will subdivide so that some of you are still practicing in a group member's home, and others are off somewhere else, such as a department store bathroom. On the whole, evenings and weekend mornings are good times for you to get together and practice in semi-public and public situations because rest rooms will be less crowded.

How to integrate new members into the group is clearly a very important question, because if they don't feel comfortable with the group the first time, they are unlikely to come back. The best way is for the group leader, or some other designated person, to meet with new members beforehand, explain to them how the group operates, show them how the group practices, and give them some BBS literature to read before they come to their first support group meeting. Obviously, at their first meeting, everyone should be cordial and friendly to newcomers, trying to integrate them into the group as fast as possible.

Almost all of the support groups to date have been exclusively male. This isn't surprising, given that only one out of ten people seeking treatment is female. If you know a woman who is interested in attending meetings, you should either help her find another female paruretic in the area (not easy to do yet), or try to find another woman who will act as support at group meetings. Either a friend of hers or a significant other/spouse of one of the male members will work.

Workshops

In 1998, the IPA developed a successful weekend workshop model based on the work of coauthor Joseph Himle. A list of current workshop offerings can be found at the IPA home page link. Conducted by coauthor Steven Soifer, they consist of no more than twenty participants and a trained moderator. Ideally, workshops take place in a private home where bathroom facilities are conducive to graduated exposure therapy. At times, workshops take place at a hotel, conference center, or university. They begin on Friday evenings and continue through Sunday afternoons.

While these workshops are currently run by professionals, lay people with appropriate training and liability insurance could easily lead them. There is a fine line between leading a support group and running a workshop. As more and more people recover from paruresis, we expect that some will want to move into leadership roles to help others get into recovery, too.

Below is a description of how a weekend workshop unfolds:

Friday evening: Friday evening is a little scary, a little intimidating, and ultimately a very emotional time. For many of the paruretics attending, it may be the first time they have ever disclosed to anyone that they suffer from BBS. The attendees gather and each person introduces him- or herself and then shares his or her experience of living with BBS. Some stories are humorous, some are traumatic, but all are touching. Amazingly, as each person speaks of the occasions of shame, embarrassment, fear, hurt, and pain of BBS, the stories are eerily similar. In listening to others share their tortuous stories, there is a shift from self-focus to focusing on others' feelings and experiences. Trust develops. Compassion is abundant. Understanding is universal. The moderator explains what to expect for the remainder of the weekend and the session ends for the night.

Saturday: A key component of the workshop is graduated exposure therapy, including the all-important fluid-loading. Water, tea, coffee and soft drinks are available at all times for the participants. When the attendees arrive Saturday morning, there is a short social time, during which everyone drinks a lot of liquids.

The facilitator then discusses the origins of BBS, urinary dynamics, and shares research about what is currently know about BBS. Everyone is asked to prepare a behavioral hierarchy, outlining which rest room situations provoke the least to the greatest levels of anxiety. Based on these models, the moderator then pairs participants up with "buddies" who are close in functioning to one another. The group begins graduated exposure therapy exercises as outlined in chapter 4. During this session, pee buddies will try to get in seven to ten trials of three-second stream initiation. After this session, the group meets to give progress reports. For those who have had a successful morning, there is much shared joy. For those who have been less successful, there is tremendous support. After the discussion, there is a lunch break.

The afternoon session reconvenes after lunch. Those who were successful in the morning session within the home or hotel environment, might move onto a more challenging environment (utilizing somewhat deserted public rest rooms in the hotel or in the nearby community). For those participants who feel more comfortable continuing where they are, the exercises continue as they did in the morning session. At the conclusion of the afternoon session, the group again meets to discuss everyone's progress before breaking for the night.

Sunday: As with Saturday, the Sunday session starts with fluid-loading. The facilitator reviews goals for the day's sessions. Buddies team up and continue the work they started Saturday. Depending on the environment, the last session usually occurs at a mall, an airport, or occasionally a major sporting event. Participants are *always* given the choice of whether or not to attend such public outings; there is absolutely no coercion involved, since this would defeat the purpose of the workshop. Again, how far you push yourself is always up to you. In fact, it is constantly stressed that you should *not* practice at a level at which you think you might fail, since building upon success after success is a basic principle of graduated exposure therapy. At the last discussion session, participants have the option of giving their contact information to others in the workshop, and they frequently do so.

Workshops are a wonderful opportunity to meet other paruretics who are geographically close and can be a nucleus of a support group for your area. One of the goals of the workshops, in fact, is to leave an active support group behind, and this has happened in most cases.

A workshop participant shares some thoughts:

It is difficult to explain the "magic" that happened at our workshop. There is no other word for it. Before attending, I knew that we were going to learn about BBS and do exercises that might help the bashful bladder syndrome, but I was totally unprepared for the overwhelming, genuine caring and concern that literally poured from the gathering. Listening to everyone's stories Friday night touched me and gave me a real understanding of what paruresis does to people. My own experience was met with empathy—not sympathy—and support. We laughed; we cried; we rejoiced in one another's success; we encouraged one another when success was not so easily forthcoming. Maybe our group was just full of special people, maybe our collective experience was unique, but I don't think so. By the time the weekend was over, it was as if we had shared the trenches together, so to speak, and we had a bond that was almost like family. I can honestly say that the weekend was one of the most uplifting times I have ever experienced, and I am grateful that I had the opportunity to participate. If anyone out there is debating whether or not to attend one of these workshops, all I can say is Go! Go! Go! *You will* not *be sorry. You will be better off for having gone. For me personally, it was truly a life-changing event.*

Yet another workshop participant, Sylvia, shares a detailed narrative about her success with graduated exposure therapy:

I am a forty-five-year-old female who has had a debilitating case of paruresis since I was seventeen. That's twenty-eight years of avoidance behaviors, including panic attacks in the bathroom and obsessing on when, where, and whether I was going to use the bathroom and if I would be able to perform or not. I was constantly missing out on happy times, intimate relationships, social outings, jobs I would have loved, nights on the town, going over to friends' houses, or anything you can imagine. Paruresis had controlled all of my behaviors and I had often felt life was passing me by. I had a severe case, and it was ruining my life.

For me, paruresis came on suddenly when, during two weeks at college, I was put into a bathroom situation that was extremely embarrassing to me. All of a sudden, I could not urinate in that rest room when people were waiting for me, whereas previously I had never had a problem urinating in any public or private rest room. Soon the problem spread to other rest rooms, bathrooms in people's houses, and it even got so bad that I could not go in my own home if anyone was around. I didn't know what to think—I was at a loss to know why this had happened to me and I didn't know that it was a phobia. All I knew was that I hated what was occurring and I felt as if I had no control over my body. I also felt ashamed and embarrassed, and so I kept the problem to myself. The secrecy only made it worse.

I became practically homebound due to my paruresis. I gave up hope of ever getting over this condition. In my twenties and early thirties I had been to psychiatrists, traditional therapists, behavioral therapists, and hypnotists. I had taken prescribed medication to help me relax and be able to void whenever I needed to. Nothing worked. Some tactics that were prescribed actually exacerbated the problem. No one I talked with had ever heard of the condition, much less knew how to cure or lessen it. After finally realizing (in my twenties) that I had a phobia, I tried to research it myself to find either a cure or information about it, but there was nothing in the literature. I felt completely alone and like a freak.

I think what a lot of people don't understand about paruresis is that the problem is not that you don't want to urinate because you're embarrassed or for any other reason; it's that you can't urinate. It's a subconscious experience where the sphincter muscles tighten, and no matter how full the bladder may be, urination is impossible under these circumstances. This is what is so frightening and debilitating about having this condition. And the action of urinating has to be performed several times a day! It's not something one can avoid.

I can seriously say that this took precedence over almost everything I did. Just the thought of having a full bladder and not being able to empty it, the fear of the pain, and of not being able to tell anyone what my problem was, scared me out of trying different things and going places. Holding urine in can be extremely unhealthy, uncomfortable, and painful, and sometimes I felt as if my bladder would burst. I would clock events—if they were going to last longer than three hours, I wouldn't attend. I used many tactics to find private rest rooms where I could void. My whole life revolved around this phobia and figuring out when and where I was going to be able to empty my bladder.

When it got to the point where I could no longer go anywhere, I decided that I had to do something about it. My therapist had found the term "paruresis" in a medical journal in 1998. I got on the Internet and looked up paruresis. I found a site called "The International Paruresis Association." You cannot believe how happy and frightened I was to have found this site. I read everything in it. Knowing that there were others who understood how I felt, and that there was help out there, comforted me. It helped to know what everyone else was going through and that I wasn't alone.

After a few months, I attended a paruresis workshop in Los Angeles, led by Steve Soifer. The workshop lasted from Friday night until Sunday afternoon. I lived nearby, and so I could go home at night. I was happy about this, because it meant I would have a "way out" if I couldn't urinate all day at the workshop. My fear has always been that I would be trapped with nowhere to go. What I didn't realize before I went to the workshop was that Steve had it set up so that no one would be or feel "trapped." He made sure there were plenty of bathrooms around, and that there were some private ones. I felt so comfortable there, I didn't have to leave, even though I could have.

Since I'm female, and it seems that the affliction occurs more frequently in men, I was the only woman paruretic at the workshop. This posed a problem, because we need "buddies" to help us with the desensitization therapy. There were seven men at the workshop, and fortunately for me, one man had brought along his wife (a non-paruretic) who agreed to be my buddy. She was kind, non-demanding, and non-judgmental, and she helped me tremendously.

On Friday night, I arrived at the hotel and found that most of the other members of the workshop were already there, sitting around in a circle in the hotel room. I had known I would be the only woman at the workshop, but seeing the group of men intimidated me. I seriously did not want to be talking about my problem with these male strangers. Steve greeted me, introduced me to everyone, and I started feeling a little more comfortable. Also, my female "buddy" was there, and I met her, so that made me feel more relaxed, too.

Friday evening, Steve talked about BBS and told us how we were going to proceed. He also said that he was a therapist and a recovering paruretic and that he would be participating in the workshop with us. I couldn't believe someone had the strength to sit there and tell us that he couldn't pee in public, was trying to find a cure, and was going to "practice" with us. He didn't seem ashamed of having the phobia, which *helped me tremendously. I realized that maybe I wasn't so weird after all, that maybe my problem was partly physical and so it wasn't completely my fault for being so inadequate. I also realized that it was possible to have BBS and not hate myself, feel ashamed, lonely, inadequate, helpless, and fearful. I envisioned the possibility of an acceptance of my problem in tandem with the possibility of curing it. What I realize now is that acceptance is crucial to recovery. But acceptance of paruresis had never occurred to me until that first evening of the workshop.*

For the rest of the evening, all of us in the group told our stories about what it was like living a life with paruresis. The stories were very similar to my own: the same avoidance patterns, the same fears, the same frustrations, the same reasons for not being able to urinate in certain rest rooms (such as they are too quiet and someone might hear, or that someone is waiting). The way BBS began was different for everyone, it seemed, but it would eventually manifest itself in the same ways.

Some had more severe problems than others. We rated ourselves at the beginning of the workshop as to how severe we each thought our phobia was and how much it affected our lives.

The next morning we came back to the hotel prepared to practice desensitization all day. We all brought large quantities of bottled water, or soda (which isn't the best choice, since it has caffeine in it, a stimulant) or juice. We drank and talked until we had to "go." I made sure I didn't have to go right when I got there. But with all the liquid in me, soon my bladder was full, and the urge to void could not be delayed.

I have a problem even telling people or letting people know that I am going to the bathroom. When we started the desensitization therapy, I had a difficult time, but finally I got up without saying anything and went into the bathroom in the other room. To be honest, I can't remember if I voided or not; I just remember that getting up and actually going into the dreaded place with people knowing what I was doing was an accomplishment.

Then we started out on the real work. The men went their own ways—some into different hotel rooms to practice with a partner, some stayed in that hotel room. There was a private bathroom down the hall in case a person needed full privacy without anyone around, and so we had an "out" if we needed it. A few other people and I used it several times.

The idea behind desensitization is not to proceed any faster than you think you can. We had each written down our hierarchies of various bathroom situations, the easiest first, and then up to the most difficult, last. We would start with the easiest, and then when that was accomplished with success, we would go on to the next. I think this is what worked so well in the program. I never felt totally panicked in a situation that I was in.

My buddy, Margie, walked with me up to her hotel room. We went inside and looked at it and talked for a while. She showed me the bathroom. I looked inside with fear. So I was going to have to pee in there with her around? It seemed impossible. I shook my head. "Uh, uh," I told her. "Nope. You're going to have to wait down the hall."

Even though Margie was at the end of the hall, I closed the hotel door room and locked it. I wanted to make sure she wasn't coming in. Then I went into the bathroom and locked that door. At first I started to feel my heart race a little and I felt some panic coming on. But then I realized that no one was coming in, there was no need to hurry, and if I couldn't go, I always had the option of saying so and trying again there or somewhere else. It was no longer a secret. This was the greatest relaxant in the world.

The way that Steve said to practice desensitization, so that we could learn to use the sphincter muscle and be able to urinate several times in a row without having to hydrate ourselves again, was to urinate for three seconds, and then stop. This is considered a success because often it is the starting of the urination process that is the most difficult. Of course, after only three seconds, the bladder would still be full, but then I would be able to practice again a few minutes later. Also, the desensitization techniques included the practice that if we were in the bathroom and couldn't urinate within two minutes (I gave myself five), we were to stop, go out, and then try again later. Otherwise the tension would build up and it would make things worse.

I was successful on the first attempt, after only a minute or two. I went down the hall to Margie, and she was very happy for me. Next, I had Margie move one foot closer, and I had yet another successful attempt at voiding.

My buddy and I continued with this procedure for the next two hours. Slowly, foot by foot, she would come closer down the hallway, stand and read her book, while each time I would go inside the hotel room and close both doors, then use the bathroom. It worked every time. I got used to her being closer and I knew exactly where she was; she totally respected my space and did what I asked her to do. She was also very supportive and told me I could do it. I was starting to feel elated.

Then she was standing right outside the hotel room door, with the door closed. I went into the hotel room, closed the bathroom door, urinated for three seconds, and then came out. She was getting very near my "danger zone." The next step was to leave the hotel room open. We did that while she stood outside the door and read her book. I closed the bathroom door—and success again. I then had her stand outside the open door and not read her book, but just wait for me. That was hard, because I kept thinking that she was thinking about me, but she really wasn't, and so I went. Success again.

If we had started out on our sojourn with her standing right outside the open hotel door, I never would have been able to urinate in the bathroom. But the slow steps, and knowing that I was in charge of myself and that she respected my space and felt empathy for my situation, encouraged me and fostered improvement.

Then for the big step: She came inside the hotel room with me. I asked her to stand near the window and read her book while I used the rest room with the door closed. She did, and I went, and it was great. Then slowly, step by step, and foot by foot, she came closer each time, until she was sitting on a chair very close to the bathroom door. I knew she could hear me, but I told myself it was all right. I started to feel nervous, but I urinated for three seconds and came out overjoyed.

Then there was a problem. Margie moved her chair one foot closer and touched the outside wall of the bathroom with her fingers. "See?" she said. "I'm so close I can touch it now. You're really doing great." That did it. I knew I wouldn't be able to go. She had touched the bathroom wall, and so, in my mind, had crossed my comfort zone of proximity. I felt deflated. I asked her not to touch the wall, but it was too late. I went into the rest room and tried for about three or four minutes but gave up. I knew it was impossible. I couldn't go, simply because she had touched the bathroom wall. It was the only time I felt she had invaded my space and I knew that she had done it inadvertently. She had had no idea of how it would affect me.

The good thing was that I could come out and tell her I

couldn't go, and why. I asked her to move her chair backwards a couple of feet. This gave me the space I needed. I went into the bathroom and voided completely. This was possible for me only because, in my mind, she was two feet farther away from me, and that made all the difference. She hadn't crossed my invisible line.

After this, we went back to the workshop hotel room where many of the other participants had gathered. We all talked about our experiences, successes, and some disappointments. I was beginning to feel a "shift" in my brain that hadn't occurred for decades. I can't quite explain it, but something was telling my subconscious, "It's okay, it's safe."

After lunch, we started practicing again. In the hotel room, Margie stood back farther than she had the previous time, although she was still in the room. Sometimes she read her book; sometimes she just sat there. She slowly came closer and didn't touch the wall, as I had asked her not to do. Finally, she was sitting in her chair directly in front of the bathroom. It was quiet, but I turned on the light and the fan. I felt she was very close, but I still felt safe enough to go, and was successful again. Then I thought I would try it without the fan on. This meant that not only could she hear me urinate, but I could hear that she was there, turning the pages of her book, making rustling movements in her chair. This is what causes the adrenaline rush—the hypersensitivity to sights and sounds and obsessive thoughts. But I was able to overcome them, and I urinated in a quiet bathroom with a woman friend sitting right outside! This had not happened in years.

At the end of the day, the group met and again told our stories of the day's desensitization process. Margie also related how she felt while she was helping me and how she really wasn't thinking about what I was doing. That was a revelation to me, because I always thought that everyone was so concerned about what I was doing in the bathroom. I know now that that is a fallacy, and in truth, everyone is basically concerned with him- or herself, and no one is thinking about my bathroom habits one bit. Also, it's nobody's business what I'm doing in there. I don't have to report or explain what I'm doing or did in the bathroom, unless I want to.

I guess desensitization is partly a matter of "toilet assertiveness training." I needed to learn how to stand my ground in the bathroom and not let others—or my thoughts about what others are thinking—deter me from getting my needs met. I learned at this workshop that I could claim my space and I had a right to it.

On Sunday, we met in the morning. This time, instead of staying in the hotel room, we went out to a mall that was nearby. Margie first stood outside the rest room, a distance away. I was successful in voiding. Then she came closer to the closed door. The difference this time was that someone else came into this very quiet bathroom. I was successful again while this unknown woman was there! I know she heard me urinate, but I didn't care, and I'm sure she didn't either. It is much easier for me to urinate around people I don't know, but not always possible, so this was also a success.

Then, for a major test. Margie came into the rest room with me. At first we just stood and talked for a few minutes. This was a desensitization process in itself for me because I had not gone into the bathroom willingly with anyone I knew for years. And I had not urinated in a rest room with anyone I knew for decades. After we talked, I asked her to wash her hands or run the water and not think about me. I went to the end stall, and it took a couple of minutes, but I urinated. I felt amazed at what two days of practice could do for me, after twenty-eight years of suffering from this phobia.

We went into another rest room in a department store. This rest room was a little bit busy. I don't like people waiting for my stall or talking loudly (it makes me nervous), so this was a test. Also, Margie was in the rest room with me, standing on the other side of the room. I went into a stall and urinated while people were waiting for my stall. I couldn't believe it. I felt better about myself with each success. Then, Margie said she had to use the toilet, so she used one several stalls away from me. I could go also. Total progress.

And now, what to me was the grand finale: Margie sat in the stall next to me and used the bathroom, while I urinated in the stall right next to her and while other people were waiting for me. This was total success for me, completely unheard of. I want to reiterate that I had not urinated with a person I knew in a stall next to me in the rest room since I first abruptly acquired the phobia of paruresis when I was seventeen. It had been twenty-eight years since I had been able to urinate with anyone I knew in the next stall. Yet, after only two days of desensitization therapy, I was able to do so. I was ecstatic, incredulous, and profoundly moved. I think I cried a little bit out of relief. I now knew that I could get over this problem.

I decided to stop while I was ahead, and in fact, I had reached my goal. To be able to urinate while someone I knew was in the rest room was my goal for the workshop, and I had achieved it. I felt as if I could do anything.

We went back to the hotel room at the end of the day and the group again shared their therapy experiences. All had improved, some more than others. But I'm sure that every person at the workshop left feeling as if they accomplished something they didn't know that they could do. It was a great feeling.

I think the workshop was so successful because it emphasized graduated exposure therapy, everyone understood and empathized with each other, and no pressure was put on anyone. There was also a "way out" if anyone needed it. Everyone knew that they would not get stuck with no where to go. Steve Soifer is also a great facilitator, very compassionate and understanding, even more so because he has suffered with the problem, too. I have also joined a support group since then, but still have not found a female buddy in my area with whom to practice.

I have relapsed somewhat since the workshop due to lack of desensitization practice. But I practice sometimes with the support group, and sometimes on my own just going to malls and into situations I wouldn't have tried before. I'm also not afraid to go anywhere anymore, because through the IPA I have found an absolute "way out" if nothing else succeeds. I use an intermittent catheter if I go somewhere and I can't urinate in the bathroom. It's discreet, gets the job done, and it gives me freedom until I am desensitized enough to be able to urinate in almost any public rest room. Just carrying the catheter gives me the feeling that I won't be stuck, so I usually don't even have to use it. I accept my disorder now, and I relish the freedom that the catheter combined with desensitization therapy has given me.

Summary

Clinical experience and a limited amount of research indicate that graduated exposure therapy is the best method to start treating BBS. If this method of treatment does not progress well and little improvement has been obtained by the tenth exposure session, additional therapies such as cognitive restructuring and applied relaxation can be added to the exposure program. If all else fails, creative solutions and self-catheterization can help paruretics manage their bashful bladder problem. Follow-up therapy is critical, group counseling and support groups are wonderfully helpful, and weekend workshops are a strong aid in the war on BBS.

Paruretics do not need to suffer. There *are* treatment options that can make life with BBS a lot more tolerable.

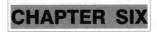

The Medical Community and Paruresis

An important step in assessing and treating paruresis is to seek medical attention from a health professional. The first medical provider you should consult is a medical doctor, such as a primary care physician, internist, or family practice doctor. The reason a medical doctor should be consulted first, as noted earlier, is that a physical cause for the inability to urinate must be ruled out before a diagnosis of bashful bladder syndrome can be made. It is important to note that most people who complain of the inability to urinate do *not* have physical conditions that are responsible for their condition.

If you are like most paruretics, the mere thought of speaking to a medical doctor about your condition will be intimidating and overwhelming. Therefore, seek out a medical professional with whom you feel comfortable talking. Rely on recommendations from family and friends or your medical insurance carrier in seeking the right doctor. If you do not feel free communicating your feelings, fears, and concerns, you have not yet found the right person. Keep looking.

After you give a history of your symptoms to your doctor and have a medical examination, the primary care physician may want to refer you to a urological specialist, or urologist, to further rule out a physical cause for the paruresis. Do not be concerned about this referral; it is a fairly common course of action. The urological system is complex and a specialist may be able to identify physiological problems of the urological system with more specificity than a family physician.

Be warned, however, that many medical providers are not yet familiar with bashful bladder syndrome as a cause for the inability to urinate. Therefore, do not assume that all urologists know of this condition and know how to treat it. It will be up to you, the patient, to be your own advocate in discussing the seriousness of paruresis in your life. We recommend that you call the urologist prior to making an appointment and indicate that you suspect bashful bladder syndrome may be the root of your inability to urinate. Rely on your own sense of comfort with the response you receive and then decide whether you feel the doctor would be open and sympathetic to such a diagnosis. It is sad to say, but because doctors' understanding of this subject varies so widely you cannot assume that you will be listened to and taken seriously. If you have any feelings of uneasiness or discomfort with the response you receive from the doctor, keep looking for another doctor.

When a physical cause for the inability to urinate has been eliminated, the search for answers will often lead to a mental health professional. There are four types of mental health professionals who might be of assistance: psychiatrists, psychologists, social workers, and counselors.

Psychiatrists specialize in treating mental health problems. While they are medical doctors and are capable of addressing the physical aspects of the problem, generally that portion of assessment is left to a urologist, as noted above. Psychiatrists can, however, prescribe medications that have been helpful with other forms of phobia. While medication alone cannot adequately address all of the dynamics of paruresis, some medications have been helpful for some patients and are worth at least investigating.

Another therapy that may be offered by a psychiatrist is behavioral therapy. Not all psychiatrists are trained in this methodology, so it may be helpful to contact the Anxiety Disorders Association of America or the Association for Advancement of Behavior Therapy for a referral.

Psychologists, social workers, and counselors are mental health professionals trained in the assessment and treatment of mental health disorders, including anxiety disorders and phobias. They are also well trained in behavioral therapy and can be helpful in assessing and treating bashful bladder syndrome.

The Doctor Visit

Once you have located a health professional with whom you feel comfortable, you may find yourself educating them. This condition has not received the attention in medical circles that it requires or deserves, which means you may be in the unfortunate position of having to educate the very person you have sought for help. Do not be intimidated by this prospect. Take your time to provide detailed information about how the inability to urinate has affected your life. Give examples of avoiding sporting events, movies, concerts, family vacations, relationship issues. Stress how extreme urgency has *no* bearing on your ability to go. Most health professionals, whether medical providers or mental health providers, will be surprised at this, erroneously believing that ultimately the physical need to urinate will overcome mental difficulties associated with not urinating. Relate one or two of the most extreme examples of situations where you were unable to urinate and the effect it had *on you*. Did you lose out on a job opportunity because you could not provide a drug test sample? Did you miss a family gathering because it was too far from your home and a safe bathroom? These are the kind of anecdotes that will help medical providers understand the enormous scope of the problem. Challenge medical providers to put themselves in your position and to think of what day-to-day activities would be restricted or impossible if they had to cope with this condition, as you have had to do on a daily basis.

The important goal during this office visit—whether at your initial medical provider's office or as you continue your process with a urologist or mental health professional—is to maintain a non-threatening, collaborative tone to facilitate the exchange of information. Remember that information on this subject was not a large part, if any part, of their training, so you cannot fault them for lacking information. Once they are aware of the underlying concepts of this phobia, they will be able to refer to treatment modalities that they know respond to this problem. Mention that you are aware that behavioral therapy has been helpful with this type of phobia. Share this book with your medical professional. Provide copies of the literature prepared by the International Paruresis Association. Your objective should be to impart important information about your condition, in order to help you conquer this problem. Communication is the key. It is not about who knows more about paruresis.

Another important goal to remember when speaking with your health provider is to be specific about the actual urinary dysfunction. Can you initiate a urine stream at home? Is the stream steady when you have privacy? Do you have the sensation of an empty bladder after completing urination? Do sights or sounds bother you? Use the self-test in chapter 1 as a checklist for the physician or mental health professional. Do not forget to mention that paruresis makes it virtually impossible to provide a urine sample for marketplace drug testing, so you need to document your inability to urinate on demand in case this issue comes up in the future. This will lay the groundwork for the possibility of an accommodation to random drug testing. Without medical documentation of your bashful bladder, the veracity of your position is compromised. It may be possible that having a note from your doctor will allow the testing facility to make alternative arrangements for the drug testing, such as blood or saliva testing. State laws vary on this issue, so there is no absolute answer, but the first line of defense is medical documentation. That is why it is crucial you speak openly, candidly, and fully about the implications of your particular situation with your health care provider. Do not sugarcoat the issue.

I Can't Bring Myself to Talk to My Doctor about Paruresis

It is all well and good for us to list what you "should" talk to your doctor about, but that presumes you are able to bring yourself to talk about this embarrassing problem. We are aware of how difficult that thought is, especially to those who have suffered with this problem in silence and isolation for years and years.

The number one reason most paruretics will not discuss this problem with anyone, including medical providers, is *fear*. Fear is a very powerful emotion that can grip our hearts and choke the words right out of our throats. The most common fears paruretics suffer are fear of being judged negatively, fear of being laughed at, fear of being viewed as less of a person (for men, less masculine), fear of being dismissed, or fear of being thought crazy. These are distorted thoughts that can be greatly helped by cognitive restructuring, as outlined in chapter 5. Cognitive restructuring involves identifying inaccurate, distorted thinking and replacing those thoughts with more truthful self-statements. Reject the negative remarks and remind yourself that it is worse to continue to struggle with the problem than to risk talking about it and getting help.

A second method of managing your fear of discussing this problem with your medical provider is a technique with which you are already familiar, exposure therapy. Over time, the experience of revealing your problem to health professionals will help to reduce your fear of talking about the problem. This is the same dynamic as talking about your problem with family and loved ones—the shroud of secrecy is removed and the backbone of paruresis starts to break.

Summary

It is important, though not essential, to work hand-in-hand with a medical professional to overcome paruresis. Establishing a relationship with a medical professional includes divulging the secret of paruresis, and oftentimes educating him or her. The thought of reaching out for medical help with shy bladder syndrome is a daunting proposition, which relaxation techniques and cognitive restructuring can help. Sometimes, even after you summon the courage to talk to a doctor, he or she does not respond favorably. If this happens, you must remind yourself that not all doctors are the same; they are people, too. If you are having trouble communicating with the medical provider you've found, don't waste your time. Move on. Tell the next provider that you felt the need to seek out another physician because you were not listened to or taken seriously by a previous medical provider. Let them know up front that you expect respect, that you are seeking help, and that you are your own health care advocate.

Take control of your paruresis and it will cease to control you.

CHAPTER SEVEN

How Family Members, Intimate Partners, and Friends Can Support Your Recovery

To someone who has never experienced BBS, it may not appear to be that big of a deal. What does it matter if someone can't urinate in public? It's not like having a disease or an addiction, right? Wrong. The truth is, living with BBS is nothing short of a nightmare from which you never wake up. It is impossible to avoid the problem, simply as a function of the physical necessity of daily voiding.

A forty-year-old woman tells the story of how she learned of her boyfriend's lifelong struggle with paruresis:

> He closed his eyes and leaned his head back against the front seat of the car. Then he said, "I have something to tell you. When I tell you, it will make total sense of my ways. It will explain everything." He let out a big sigh, in obvious pain and distress. I wondered what could be so huge, so difficult, so awful for him to tell me? Had he been abused as a child? Did he have an addiction problem with drugs or alcohol? He turned to me and said, "I have this problem. I've had it for the last twenty-five years. I can't pee in public places. You're the first person I've ever told in my life."
>
> My first reaction, before all the implications of that statement had sunk in, was that this was not as bad as I feared, even if it obviously was traumatic for him. Initially, I

was relieved. He continued, "That's why I don't go out much, why I don't like to drive long distances. I can use my bathroom at my apartment most of the time, but when you're there, it's hard sometimes. I dropped out of school in ninth grade because I couldn't go to the bathroom at school. When I went back to college after getting my GED, it was to a local college so that I could be close to my bathroom at home. The experience of going away to college was never an option."

It was then that my mind began to race to previous situations: The first time we went to the movies he wanted to go to the theater that was a block away from his place, even though nothing good was playing. He had said he was going to spend all day with my kids and me, but he left after only a few hours. He never drank much when we went out, alcohol or otherwise. He had refused to travel with me to a wedding that was two hours away. He was reluctant to change jobs, even though he detested his present job and had the credentials and schooling to get a much better position.

I had chalked up these behaviors—and many others—to his unique idiosyncrasies. I never could have imagined the reason for it all. But once I knew about it, I couldn't imagine living with anything worse.

Unfortunately, this man's experience is a common one for paruretics. In some form or fashion, BBS dictates where you work, the type of social life you have (or, more to the point, do not have), how you interact in relationships, travel (or, lack of it), and how you relate to your family. It affects every aspect of your life. There is no vacation away from having to urinate. There is nowhere to hide from the problem. There is precious little information in the public about BBS, let alone sympathy. No celebrity has yet to come forward and proclaim that he or she has BBS, rallying public support, funding, and research. And, sadly, as a result of the lack of information and sensitivity to this problem, there are currently very few resources available to help people who suffer with BBS.

The simple truth is, without intervention and treatment, BBS can—and does—destroy lives.

The Impact on Spouses, Family Members, and Significant Others

It is indisputable that it is the paruretic who suffers the most from BBS. Yet, family members and significant others suffer as well. Just as there are few support options for paruretics themselves, there is nowhere for loved ones to turn.

Since many paruretics choose not to divulge their condition, it is common for loved ones to be kept in the dark. This secret can continue for years and years. If you are close to a paruretic but are ignorant of their condition, your loved one or family member's behavior may seem bizarre, irrational, and hurtful. A father who will not take his son to a baseball or football game; a mother who will not take her daughter to the mall; a spouse who will not eat out or attend any cultural events; a child who will only consider a college that is within a short distance of home; a family member who refuses to go on vacation: All are exhibiting behavior typical of BBS.

Because the paruretic will not divulge the real reason behind this behavior, the unknowing partner to the condition incorrectly— and understandably—attributes the behavior to other reasons: "She doesn't like my family, so she refuses to travel to spend the holidays at my parents' house"; "If my dad really loved me more than he did his work, he would take me to see the Yankees play"; "Our son is tied to his mother's apron strings, he just won't go away to school. I don't think he will ever leave home."

It is also common for resentment and hurt to build over the years to the degree that relationships are strained, or do not survive. The paruretic is left with nothing; the loved one has nothing either, not even an understanding of why.

Dating someone with paruresis can be confusing and painful if you don't know what's going on.

We were having a wonderful evening at my place. He had suggested that we stay in, so I had fixed a really nice dinner. After dessert and coffee, we began to be romantic. It was great. All of a sudden, he just got up and left. No explanation, no nothing, he just mumbled something about having to leave. He hasn't called me since. I thought we were having a lovely time and were really getting along. I guess he didn't care about me after all. Either that, or he was just one more jerk.

How can loved ones understand when they are unaware of the existence of the problem? How do you fight a shadow?

For paruretics, the guilt of not being able to perform the "normal" task of urinating in public is further compounded by the guilt that results from leaving a trail of misperceptions. Paruresis colors every decision in your life, so it cannot help but impact those around you. It is yet one more horrible component of suffering with BBS that you would rather allow people to think negatively of you than reveal what the issue really is about. It hurts less to let other people think you're "just one more jerk" than to tell the truth.

If you can gather the courage—and make no mistake, it takes courage—to inform loved ones of the problem, you may be pleasantly surprised at their reaction. The knowledge that what appears to be unreasonable behavior on your part has a genuine cause—a cause that has nothing to do directly with them—is a tremendous relief. It makes rational that which appeared to be totally irrational. It is no longer a fight against a shadow; it is a fight against an identifiable problem. It is quite common at this point for paruretics to seek professional help for their problem, often at the urging of their family member or significant other. Armed with support, love, and understanding, seeking help is not as daunting a task.

After telling a loved one, however, paruretics often feel embarrassed at divulging their secret. It is a critical time, during which paruretics need understanding, caring, and concern, but *not pity*. Fear of being seen in a weak light or perceived as a freak by loved ones fuels a paruretic's decision to keep it a secret.

The following story is typical:

> *I am living at home with my mom and dad. I am able to go freely when they are around the house—they are the only ones I feel comfortable going around. I fear that if I tell either of them, I will have a feeling in my mind that they are always listening for me struggling after that, and I might lose the ability to go around them. It is hard to explain this thought since it is irrational and illogical, yet emotionally real.*

Sometimes, the paruretic will not face the problem. If he or she does not want to address the problem, there is little a loved one can do:

> *In twenty-five years of having BBS, I was the first person he ever told. I felt honored that he trusted me enough to tell me, but looking back, that was the beginning of the end of our dating relationship. He just could not handle the thought that in my mind he was less of a man because he had this problem. I didn't feel that way at all—quite the contrary, I marveled at all he had accomplished in his life while accommodating this horror. But, in the end, he decided he would rather live alone with his problem than face it with me. There was nothing I could do.*

Finding Out a Loved One Has Paruresis—What Do You Do?

So, if you are a family member or significant other, how can you help the paruretic once you are told? The most important thing you can do is not be judgmental about paruresis. Listen carefully to what the paruretic has experienced, is feeling, the fears he or she has. Do not minimize the condition. Recognize and acknowledge the courage it took to share such a devastatingly embarrassing secret. Be open. Be compassionate. Do *not* be condescending and by all means do *not* exhibit pity. The paruretic needs affirmation that your good opinion has not changed by learning this information. Give it freely and give it often. In addition, you can aid the recovery process by functioning as a buddy in treatment (explained in chapter 4), and by being available to listen.

Because the subject of paruresis is sensitive on many levels, it is helpful to allow paruretics to determine when it is talked about and to what extent. Otherwise, they may begin to obsess that you only see them in light of the paruresis. This perpetuates obsessive thinking and is counterproductive to the support that is so crucial during recovery.

Remember: You may well be the first person the paruretic has told about the problem, perhaps in their entire life. Your reaction could have a tremendous effect, good or bad, on whether or not the they feel they can tell others or seek medical treatment. If you react with ridicule or mockery, the paruretic will clam up for good, perpetuating the secrecy and abandoning behaviors that would lead to a cure. If, however, you react with kindness and sensitivity, their worst fears of being judged will dissipate and a healthy approach to treatment may begin.

Summary

Family members, intimate partners, and friends can play a vital and important role in the paruretic's recovery from BBS. Understanding and embracing the enormity of the impact of paruresis on your loved one's life, being compassionate and nonjudgmental, listening, and allowing the paruretic to direct the flow of information on the subject, are all ways to support the paruretic in the struggle to overcome this condition.

CHAPTER EIGHT

Evolving Legal Ramifications: The Americans with Disabilities Act and Mandatory Drug Testing

While just being paruretic causes daily suffering, there are also some legal ramifications to consider. Mandatory drug testing is a major issue for paruretics. The "pee on demand" requirement of mandatory drug testing, whether for hiring, ongoing employment, or prison drug-testing purposes, is beyond the physical capability of paruretics. Thus, the failure to produce a urine specimen on demand can have grave consequences.

Clearly, people with BBS need some accommodation. So far, though, the Americans with Disabilities Act, or ADA, is the only piece of legislation that paruretics can hope to invoke as a basis for discrimination litigation.

The Americans with Disabilities Act

The Americans with Disabilities Act, enacted in 1990, grew out of the Rehabilitation Act of 1973, which addressed the issue of discrimination against employees within the federal government. The purpose of the ADA was to extend the protection provided for disabled citizens to the private sector.

While the intent of the ADA is worthy, it is important to note that the scope of the law is still being tested in the courts. To date, no clear test case of discrimination due to paruresis has been brought before the courts. It is inevitable that this will change; but for now, a paruretic who succeeds in a discrimination suit under the ADA would be making new law. The ADA is a complicated piece of legislation; if you are contemplating invoking the protection of the ADA with regard to your paruresis, you should consult an attorney.

The ADA provides the definition of a person with a disability as a person who:

A. Has a physical or mental impairment that substantially limits one or more of the individual's major life activities;

B. Has a record of such impairment; or

C. Is regarded as having such an impairment. (29 U.S.C. Section 706(8)A)(Rehabilitation Act); 42 U.S.C. Section 12102(2) (ADA).)

How might this apply to paruretics? First, the courts have held that a mental impairment is protected under the ADA if it is a mental or psychological disorder recognized by generally accepted medical authorities, to wit, the *DSM-IV*. Examples of mental impairments that have been held to fall under the protection of the ADA include depression (*Pesterfield* v. *Tennessee Valley Authority*, 941 F.2d 437 6th Cir. 1991) and obsessive-compulsive disorder (*Kerno* v. *Sandoz Pharmaceuticals Corp.*, 4 A.D. Cases 1195 N.D. Ill. 1989). Secondly, it is a requirement that there be a *record of such impairment*. This provision makes it crucial to seek and obtain medical documentation of paruresis. An action under the ADA could not be brought without such documentation.

Among other things, the ADA defines discrimination on the basis of disability in employment. With regard to paruresis, the critical provisions of what constitutes discrimination are: "[F]ailing to make reasonable accommodations to allow disabled persons to perform in the workplace; and using selection criteria, standards or tests that screen out or tend to screen out an individual or class of individuals with a disability" (42 U.S.C. Section 12112 [b] [5] and [6]).

"Failing to make reasonable accommodations" for paruretics could apply to the failure to supply optional bathroom facilities as well as the failure to provide alternative methods of drug testing. The practice of only allowing urinalysis for drug testing is arguably a selection criteria or test which screens out paruretics—if you cannot provide a urine sample for drug testing, you are certainly *not* selected and *are* screened out of an applicant pool.

Yet another criteria of the ADA is that an ADA lawsuit cannot be brought until *after* the employee has filed a claim with the Equal Employment Opportunity Commission (EEOC). When an individual files an EEOC claim, the employer is put on notice that there is a dispute, and the nature of the dispute is disclosed. There are specific rights and remedies under the EEOC. Since an EEOC claim must be filed prior to the institution of an ADA action, the ADA inherently requires that an employer be made aware of what the nature of the disability is, in order for the suit to go forward. If the employee has not divulged the disability, whether on a job application or even during the course of verbal interaction with a superior, the employer cannot be held accountable for having discriminated against the employee.

Mandatory Drug Testing

Employment drug testing is one of the greatest life issues facing paruretics today. For those paruretics seeking any job that requires a pre-hire drug urinalysis, the choice is either to divulge that they have BBS to a potential employer (which is not really a choice given the secrecy that a paruretic typically possesses about his or her BBS) or pass up the opportunity. Considering the steady increase of employers who require mandatory drug testing, employment opportunities for paruretics are narrowing. Said one paruretic:

> *I've had paruresis since I was probably twelve to fourteen? I don't really remember when it started, but I know that it's gotten progressively worse since I entered college. . . . I think that I first remember the early signs of this problem after failing to produce urine samples for my doctor. This first happened when I was thirteen. Since this time I have been unable to produce urine samples, and this is the one thing I greatly dread, considering that I will be graduating in May and will undoubtedly be asked to take a drug test for whatever job I am offered.*

How Employment Drug Testing Evolved

Prior to the 1980s, drug testing in the marketplace was rare. For an overview of its recent history, we went to Don Shatinsky, who works for the U.S. Department of Transportations, Drug and Alcohol Policy Office. According to Shatinsky (1999), drug testing has it roots in the "war on drugs" started by the Reagan administration in the late 1980s. During this time the U.S. Department of Labor developed workplace drug-testing guidelines. The result was the Drug Free Workplace initiative, written primarily for government and industry. What is important to realize is that these were guidelines, to be implemented by workplaces only if they so desired. They did *not* mandate random drug testing, which is the norm today. So, what changed?

During 1989 to 1990, there were a series of serious transportation-related accidents, in particular one in Maryland and one in New York, that received national attention. The New York accident involved the driver's use of marijuana and alcohol. As a result, Congress passed the Omnibus Transportation Employee Testing Act of 1991, mandating pre-hire and random drug testing for *all* employees at the federal, state, and local governmental levels *and in* private industries who were involved in transportation related work.

The regulations developed by the Department of Transportation (DOT) that would govern drug testing for the workplace became known as Part 40 of the Code of Federal Regulations (CFR). Part 40 also specifies that employers who have more than $100,000 in federal contracts must certify that they have a drug free workplace.

DOT regulations were challenged in the state of Connecticut and were upheld as meeting the constitutional test. Consequently, many employers, both in the public and private sectors, felt confident in adopting the DOT regulations. Many states do not allow random drug testing, however, since it (1) is perceived as an infringement on the Fourth Amendment (search and seizure), and (2) many jobs at the state, county, and city levels (not to mention in private industry) are not safety sensitive. Even in those states, though, federal guidelines are in place for safety sensitive industries, such as transportation by truck, rail, or air.

The Urinalysis Requirement

Since DOT regulations are used by many private as well as public employers, it is helpful to understand why the DOT requires a urinalysis and not some other method in testing for drug use. Urinalysis is the lab test of choice, primarily due to the standardization of certified testing sites. Over seventy labs use the same technology, as certified by the DOT. Blood, hair, saliva, catheterization, and patch testing procedures are not currently certified by the DOT. While the

Department of Health and Human Services is currently looking at alternatives, none of them meet DOT standards.

Cost is also a factor. A urine test may cost in the neighborhood of $5–10 per employee; other procedures might cost four to five times that amount. It is important to recognize that employees do *not* have the option to request an alternative form of testing under DOT regulations, even if you offer to pay for it out of your own pocket.

How DOT Testing Is Performed

DOT regulations require that there be a split specimen. Bathroom privacy *is* permissible. An employee or potential employee is required to ingest 42 fluid ounces (one quart, 10 ounces) of water and is then given up to three hours to produce a 45 milliliter sample. Of course, the collector hangs around during this period of time, but has much discretion as to how much privacy to grant the testee.

Importantly, if you cannot produce a sample, you can request a medical exam. If the doctor excuses you for any reason, the test is canceled. However, and this is the key for paruretics, *situational anxiety is not a defense, unless there is prior documentation*. So what is the practical significance here? It would seem that the only medical excuse you could get from a doctor would be for a physical problem, such as an enlarged prostate. Psychological causes would appear to be ruled out as an excuse, unless your medical or psychiatric history shows otherwise. This puts paruretics, who loathe disclosing their condition to anyone in a double bind.

If you are caught trying to smuggle in an old specimen, DOT regulations then allow for another specimen to be collected under direct observation. Moreover, if you test positive—or negative but with a diluted specimen—your employer has the option of testing you again under direct observation.

Among other things, the ingestion of so much water within such a short time is potentially medically hazardous. For severe paruretics whose job could be on the line, random drug testing procedures can feel like torture. We would suggest to paruretics who get randomly tested, and fail because they are unable to produce a sample, that they get tested under safer conditions at their private physician's office that very same day.

It must be noted that except in certain limited situations, the law does *not* require employers to do drug tests. Having such procedures could be costing employers excellent applicants who will not apply for jobs with firms who do drug testing.

DOT Regulations in the Year 2000— Changes Are Coming

In early 2000, the DOT issued a Notice of Proposal for Rule Making (NPRM) for Part 40 of the CFR. It has been ten years since the first rules were introduced, and the government recognized a need to incorporate new interpretations, as well as the need to put the rules in simpler terms. The public had 120 days to respond to the DOT's notice. DOT officials were looking for input in several areas, including paruresis. In particular, they wanted proposed solutions to the problem and comments from organizations like the IPA. The IPA made several suggestions, including limiting the fluid intake to no more than 24 ounces (for example, two cans of soda), and decreasing the time limit to two hours when conducting drug testing in the workplace. Furthermore, if someone were to be subject to random drug testing, and claimed to have shy bladder syndrome, then immediate alternative testing procedures would be allowed, for example, blood, hair, saliva, patch, or catheterization. The fact that someone is willing to engage in an alternative test to urinalysis, on the spot, would be an indication of good faith. The bottom line is that there *must* be a loosening in the presumption that the failure to produce a urine specimen by voiding is equivalent to a refusal to cooperate.

Beyond the DOT: Drug Testing in the Private Sector

The DOT's recommendations quickly caught on with private sector employers who were looking for ways to minimize the economic impact of drugs in the marketplace. By screening workers for drug usage, employers would then theoretically be able to identify employees or potential employees who had drug problems that could potentially affect productivity and work safety.

Many employers now require pre-hire drug screening with a urine test. How much privacy is afforded varies. In some cases, the observer may personally witness the urine passing from the body into the specimen collection cup. This is *not* required, except in the case of someone who has failed the test before. Since being watched while urinating is one of a paruretic's biggest fears, most paruretics will avoid interviewing with companies that require a pre-screening drug urinalysis.

For those paruretics who already have a job but are subject to random drug testing, reaction to drug testing ranges from concern to outright panic. Faced with the choice to either divulge the BBS to an employer or produce a urine sample under the pressure and scrutiny of a stranger, paruretic employees typically quit, get fired, or attempt to substitute another person's urine for their sample, which, if discovered, is generally grounds for termination. Employers grow suspicious when paruretics feign illness or make up excuses rather than provide a sample.

Says one paruretic:

> *As you know, there were some public policy changes concerning employer rights to demand drug screening tests of employees. An incident at work related to this put me in a near suicidal mode, because to put it bluntly, if someone held a gun to my head and said, "Pee or I pull the trigger," I would die.*

As previously mentioned, urinalysis is not the only available method of testing for drug use. The two most common alternatives are hair analysis and blood testing. Though not mandatory, urinalysis is still the preferred method of testing because (1) it is far less expensive and (2) blood testing is an invasive procedure. While some employers will allow their employees to choose an alternative form of testing, they don't have to do so. The same holds true for allowing employees more privacy and/or time to provide a urine specimen.

Random Drug Testing in Prisons

The possibility of drug testing in the marketplace is a horrible issue for paruretics, but there is yet a worse drug-testing scenario: random drug testing in prison.

There are paruretics, within the population of prisoners, just as there are within the general population. Prison is a hellish nightmare for paruretics because of the never-ending lack of privacy. Accommodating paruresis in prison on a daily basis is difficult, if not practically impossible, but nowhere is paruresis more horrendously delineated than within the prisons' random drug testing policies and procedures.

There is no question that drug testing within prisons is a useful administrative tool to identify which prisoners are using drugs, and we do *not* advocate halting the process of random drug testing in the prisons. The requirements that the testing be random and without advance warning is unilaterally fair to all prisoners. However, the requirement that drug testing be *urinalysis or nothing* is *not* fair to all prisoners, since it is impossible for a prisoner who has BBS to urinate on demand and in the presence of a prison official.

When a prisoner cannot provide a urine sample, prison officials see it as *willfully* refusing to provide the sample, thus implying to indicate that the prisoner is using drugs. If the prisoner raises the issue of paruresis, the response is most typically that he or she is feigning the condition to avoid the testing procedures. The prisoner is then labeled a "problem case" and is written up. It is very common for prisoners to be put in solitary confinement for 60 days, lose "gain" time accrued, and in some cases, experience a loss of eligibility of parole for "refusing" to produce a urine sample for drug testing.

At least four state prison systems (Florida, Massachusetts, Maryland, and Michigan) have modified their drug testing regulations to provide accommodation for prisoners with BBS. Some of these changes came about due to actual or threatened lawsuits under the ADA on behalf of prisoners. Unfortunately, the new rules are not necessarily enforced at all levels and do not address all paruretic situations.

What Can Be Done

What can a prospective employee or prisoner with paruresis do about random drug testing?

First and foremost, anyone in one of the above situations *must* get documentation of his or her condition, particularly from a psychiatrist, psychologist, or other mental health professional who is familiar with proper *DSM-IV* coding for this condition. Ideally, the assessment and diagnosis would happen *before* a job interview or random drug test at work or during incarceration. If this is not possible, the sooner the BBS is assessed and documented, the better.

Keep in mind that while there are stigmas attached to receiving a psychiatric diagnosis, there are benefits that outweigh the embarrassment. For prospective or current employees required to produce a urine specimen for testing, you will have a stronger argument for more time, privacy, or alternative testing options if your condition is documented prior to the required testing.

The courts have not yet been presented with a clean, clear case of discrimination under the ADA due to paruresis. A psychiatric diagnosis is a requirement for claims brought under the ADA to go forward. Without the diagnosis, this issue cannot be put before the courts.

Summary

The DOT promulgated drug testing guidelines in response to transportation accidents involving the ingestion of alcohol and drugs, setting into motion the random drug testing spiral within the private sector.

Paruresis is a bona fide social phobia that should fall under the purview of the ADA's guidelines. In the absence of a test case to date, no legal protection for paruretics is afforded in the workplace, both with regard to random drug testing and bathroom accommodation. Prisoners do not have protection or alternative relief from random drug testing and are being punished and demoralized for a condition over which, absent counseling intervention, they do not have control.

For other paruretics contemplating pursuing legal action under the ADA, a claim must first be brought under the EEOC. Notice must be given of the paruresis to employers or potential employers in order to be able to pursue a claim at a later date. The secrecy dynamic of BBS prevents many paruretics from disclosing the information to anyone, let alone employers.

Prison paruretics have concerns that they will be punished if they raise the specter of their phobia within the prison system. As expected, their fear of reprisal is based on past negative experiences within the prison system.

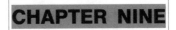

CHAPTER NINE

Future Directions

The purpose of this book has been to provide you with an overview of bashful bladder syndrome; possible causes, treatments and cures; historical perspectives on both treatment and bathroom design (see appendixes A and B); the physicality of the disorder; and legal ramifications of this condition, including the impact of random drug testing and the ADA.

However, as must be clear by now, there is much that is not known about paruresis, and in this case what we don't know *is* hurting us.

What Must Be Done

There is much to be done if more effective cures are going to be uncovered. The first step is to reach out to paruretics and let them know that they are not alone. As one anonymous writer on the paruresis bulletin board stated: "I think there are more of us than most people realize—but we're too embarrassed to admit it."

Paruresis afflicts the young with a whole lifetime ahead of them:

> *I'm seventeen and have had this disorder for most of my life. I don't think my parents know. I've hidden it from them because I'm embarrassed to talk about it. I used to think I was all alone and a weirdo for this, but I'm relieved to find that there are others like me. . . . sometimes I get so frustrated . . . I'm hoping I can overcome this phobia.*

And those who are older:

I'm 61, a retired ... journalist, happily married for almost thirty-seven years. ... I've had the problem for virtually my entire life. And until well into adulthood, I had seriously wondered if I were the only person on the planet to have it. Then I happened to read an article maybe thirty-five years ago briefly mentioning the problem. ... I was much relieved (no pun intended). ... I can identify so very closely with others' laments (problems on airplanes, worrying about sound as well as time pressure, pressure to scout out remote bathrooms, variability of difficulty in voiding even at home, etc.).

Education

There are several areas that must be addressed somewhat simultaneously. Education is a top priority. The process needs to include educating paruretics, educating the public, and educating the health care providers to this common—and treatable—anxiety disorder.

Educating Paruretics

The first step in addressing a problem is to identify it. Most paruretics do not even know there is a name for their difficulty/inability to urinate in public places. Too scared or embarrassed to talk about it, and convinced that they are the only ones who have it, they do not seek out what information is available because they do not know that their problem is real. According to one therapist:

I'm a therapist. ... I just began some marriage counseling with a couple ... the husband requested to see me privately ... his concern is avoidant paruresis ... he believes he is alone ... has trouble believing that other men have the same problem.

The paruresis Web site has provided a wealth of information to many people with BBS; however, most people stumble onto the bulletin board or are told about the Web site from a friend. While the Web site has had in excess of 100,000 hits since its independent inception in the mid-1990s, there are still many, many people suffering who either do not have access to the Internet or do not know how to find the Web site. This needs to change. Yet, for paruretics who have found the Web site, it has been a tremendous relief, as the following examples show:

> *I've just finished reading some of the material on your Web site and feel like I've just found a lifeboat full of survivors from the same nightmare. Not since my first AA meeting twenty-four years ago have I felt the same sense of camaraderie I feel reading the many letters about our problem.*

> *Earlier this evening my therapist suggested I search the Web for BBS info. And I found you! I shouldn't be surprised because I'm familiar with the scope of info on the Web, but after I read a little and answered the questions I realized I wasn't alone. Thank you for your efforts. I'm [a] thirty-one-year-old male and have been suffering with BBS for as long as I can remember. I need some new ideas and some plans for action! I have high hopes for 1997.*

> *When I first found your Web site I began to cry as I read page after page—and I don't cry easily. This problem has affected me for somewhere around six or seven years (I'm fairly fortunate compared to a lot of people, I suppose). It has at times driven me to the point of insanity ... and suicidal thoughts are never far from my mind when I think about this thing (this dragon, as one therapist put it) being incurable. But just seeing and reading things on your site has given me the hope (and some despair reading some people's posts) and encouragement to try and beat this son-of-a-*****! Thank You! Thank You!*

> *I want to thank you for having this site. I'm female and for a long time I felt that I was the only person who had this problem. I'm glad to know that I'm not. It's a pain sometimes because I just admitted my problem to my mother, who is not pee shy, and she tells me that I've got to just force myself to go and to stop telling myself that I can't go. She doesn't understand that this just doesn't help.*

> *Reading your letters section was sad and very moving. I'm struck by how many men haven't told their wives.*

> *I'm twenty-three years old and I've been dealing with BBS for about as long as I can remember (probably around age six). I didn't know until I found your site that the condition even had a name. I happened to see a movie recently in which a little boy explains that he is bladder shy, so I thought I would*

*search for it on the Internet and, lo and behold, I found your
site! I've always thought that I was weird or different because
of my problem. It's extremely, extremely nice to know that I'm
not alone.*

Educating the General Public

While, admittedly, paruretics are part of the public, it is important to equally address the issue of raising non-paruretic public
awareness to—and sensitivity, to—paruresis. As an oddity or uncommon point of discussion, reactions from people can be very negative:

"That's the dumbest thing I ever heard—everyone knows how
to go to the bathroom."

"I never heard of it. I don't know a single person who has it. If
it's so common or real, I would know."

"If they drank more, they could go. I could never hold it."

Such disbelief and lack of information reinforces the stereotype
of the "weird person" or "freak" who cannot urinate in public. When
it comes to public opinion, right or wrong, there is a herd—or, more
to the point, "heard"—mentality: If no one heard something, it's not
true; if everyone has heard of it, then it must be true. It wasn't so
long ago that sexual abuse, domestic violence, and eating disorders
were initially met with the same skepticism as paruresis—until
hordes of people came out from behind their cloak of secrecy to say,
"Yes, I was abused as a child"; "Yes, my husband/wife/parents beat
me"; "Yes, I have an eating disorder and I make myself throw up
after I eat." Unpleasant and/or personal topics "just weren't discussed." Nice people didn't talk about body parts or shameful situations. Yet, there is no denying that the number of people who have
come forward in the last twenty years to talk about "such things" is
staggering. Before, it was the proverbial elephant in the living room.
It took the courage of a Bess Myerson, the death of a Karen Carpen-
ter, to name a few, to make people stop and realize that people were
hurting, people needed understanding, people needed help.

And so it is with paruresis. This is a topic to be discussed on
talk shows, news shows, to be read about in newspaper and magazine articles. In this way, the public will learn about this problem.
Just as years ago the warning signs of anorexia were plastered in the
media, the indicia of paruresis must also be put before the public. If
paruresis is more openly discussed, paruretics will know that they
are not the only ones and will have less reservation about coming

forward, because they will know that they are not alone in their struggle. They will have information readily available as to how to get help. We can only hope that someday soon, people will know as much about paruresis as they do about other anxiety disorders such as agoraphobia, panic disorder, obsessive-compulsive disorder, and the fear of public speaking.

To this end, the National Paruresis Association, Inc., a non-profit organization, was cofounded in 1996 by one of the coauthors, Steven Soifer, and a Baltimore therapist, Carl Robbins. In 1997, the name was changed to the International Paruresis Association, primarily to reflect the increasing presence of Canadians on the board and in the membership, as well as interest from people throughout the world. IPA is comprised of a board of directors and has approximately 250 members throughout the United States, Canada, Australia, and other places. The primary mission of the IPA is education. Additionally, IPA serves as a resource center and clearinghouse.

With 17 million Americans experiencing paruresis in some form or fashion, can the public truly afford to continue to be so uninformed? How many schoolchildren drop out of school and never realize their full potential? How many wonderful employees never get hired because they cannot provide a sample for a drug test? How many prisoners get thrown in solitary instead of serving their time and moving on? At what emotional cost do we callously disregard the private, daily suffering of others?

The public needs to know about paruresis, so it can begin to understand and address the tremendous impact paruresis has on a large segment of the population. Paruretics need to know about paruresis in order to survive. Think about it: two goals worthy of the public's time and money.

In order to get the information widely disseminated, publicity efforts need to be intensified. Media coverage to date has included articles in such newspapers and magazines as the *Washington Post*, the *Los Angeles Times*, the *New York Post*, the *Toronto Sun*, the *Montreal Gazette*, *Men's Fitness* magazine, *U.S.A. Today* magazine, and *U.S.A. Today*, ABC News, *Newsweek*, and *Salon Magazine* on-line. There was also a radio show ("Sunday Rounds") on social phobia (with the emphasis on paruresis) which aired in 1997 on approximately 130 stations, reaching several hundred thousand listeners across the country. In 1998 and 1999, dozens of FM rock radio stations across the country did stories on the topic of paruresis. Also in 1999, Howard Stern discussed paruresis on his radio show with one of the coauthors, since Stern has come forward and told his listeners he suffers from this disorder.

Educating Health Care Providers

It is amazing that in a country known for being avant garde about many medical conditions, so little is known or understood about paruresis. Most general practitioners and many urologists are unfamiliar with BBS and don't know what to tell their clients. The worst response from a medical professional (other than being told you're crazy by your psychiatrist, which actually happened to one person) is to say to a paruretic: "Just get over it." Unfortunately, that is a common response. Personal prejudices can be found among medical professionals as well: "It happens to everybody once in a while, but it's not like a real problem"; "If you hold it long enough, you'll go. You'll have to. It just comes out." To that, paruretics would most probably want to scream, "No, it doesn't!"

Again, we go back to the example of the medical profession's initial reaction to anorexia. Before much was known about this conditions, anorectics were told by medical professionals: "Just eat." That was the cure—"Just eat." Today, even the average person knows that anorexia is a complex psychological condition that cannot be overcome by merely telling the anorectic to eat. How wonderful it would be to have the average person, as well the medical providers, know and understand that paruresis is a complex psychological condition that cannot be overcome by merely telling the person to "just urinate."

Understanding BBS—Considering the Possibilities

The need for continuing study of paruresis by knowledgeable professionals must continue. They need to do this through research, the use of new therapies, and by considering the possibilities of this condition "outside the box." In so doing, the following bears further consideration:

Obsessive-Compulsive Disorder Component

To the authors, it is clear that paruresis is best categorized as a social phobia. However, as explained in chapter 3, there are other theoretical conceptualizations worth considering.

From our perspective, one possible viewpoint of paruresis is to regard it as an obsessive-compulsive disorder. There is often an obsessive component to BBS, since many paruretics, either con-sciously or subconsciously, repeatedly ask themselves whether or not someone is going to come into the rest room. Or, if others are present, they ask themselves whether they will see or hear them trying to uri-nate. Hence, we might conceptualize paruresis as involving a "con-stant checking" ("Is someone going to see me?" "Is someone going to hear me?") obsession. This ties in with the authors' belief that a pri-mary cause of BBS is the fear that someone is scrutinizing the paruretics behavior (and therefore will negatively evaluate that behavior, from the paruretic's perspective). As one person wrote on the Web site:

> *I'm beginning to think our problem is more of an*
> *obsessive-compulsive problem. I find myself thinking about it*
> *all the time (obsession) and the avoidance behavior of avoiding*
> *certain bathrooms and situations is almost a compulsion. I*
> *wonder if anyone else has had this treated as an OCD (mostly*
> *with drugs, I guess?).*

Genetic Causes

Seeing BBS as a genetic problem would involve the understand-ing that each person is born with a certain gene to develop paruresis. While research seems to indicate that there is a genetic link to social phobias, given what we know, we'd be hard-pressed to say that there is a genetic cause for paruresis. Nonetheless, we think it's fair to say that there is a genetic propensity toward social phobia in general and perhaps paruresis in particular.

Biological Causes

Finally, as previously discussed, the biological perspective must be looked at. This view holds that BBS is actually a normal response. It's natural for any animal, including man, to have its bladder func-tions cut off in anxious or fearful situations as a survival mechanism. So, in actuality, those who can urinate in social situations are abnor-mal! This turns the problem on its head, reframing it as a normal response. Only through social conditioning do we learn to overcome this natural fear. This is a fascinating perspective that definitely removes the blame for BBS from clients.

Physiological Causes

There is some very recent evidence that at least some paruretics suffer from a urological disorder caused by a constricted bladder neck muscle. This new and potentially exciting discovery may mean that some people with paruresis could experience a relief in their symptoms through either a mini-transurethral resection of the prostate (TURP) or transurethral microwave therapy (TUMT). Both of these surgical procedures are used with male patients suffering from benign prostate hypertropy (BPH). At least two people with fairly severe cases of paruresis reported a 90 percent or better relief of their symptoms after this form of surgery. It must be noted that in neither case did the urologist find an actual physical obstruction in the bladder neck or urethra areas. These are controversial findings, and it is much too early to tell whether such a procedure would help other male paruretics. Moreover, these surgical procedures are *not* approved for treating paruresis. But in looking for effective treatments to help paruretics, especially severe cases, we need to keep an open mind. The future will yield more data on the effectiveness or ineffectiveness of such surgical procedures for paruresis.

Prevalence of BBS—Just How Many Have It?

Because of the recent national co-morbidity study by Kessler et al. (1997), we now know that about 6.7 percent of the population suffers from the fear of using public restrooms. However, because of the phrasing of the question in the study, we do not know how severe the problem is for people, and whether or not they are true paruretics. As a result, additional work needs to be done to identify the range of severity of paruresis in the general U.S. population. Our best conservative guess is that of the estimated 17 million people who answered this question in the affirmative, at least 10 percent would be classified as paruretics (according to *DSM-IV* criteria), and of this 1.7 million people, 10 percent of those would be classified as severe paruretics, i.e., who suffer enough from the problem that it interferes in their social and/or work life in a very significant way.

Uniform Assessment Scales for BBS

As we have seen, different assessment scales have been used over the years to ask clients questions related to BBS. For example, psychologist and coauthor Joseph Himle has developed the quick bashful bladder assessment scale (see chapter 1). We would like to see all anxiety disorder clinics, as well as medical and therapeutic professionals confronted with possible paruretic patients, use the Himle scale in order to ascertain whether or not a client has parureis. Such a uniform scale would not only be helpful in diagnosing the patient, but it would also help quantify information about paruretics that could be used in further research.

The logic of using a uniform scale is simple: If different measurements are used, it is harder to determine "how far we've come" in both diagnosis and treatment. People with BBS can fall through the cracks of diagnosis because of lack of information or education. Conversely, the Himle scale gives professionals a more objective tool for diagnosis of this elusive condition. Patients would have a higher confidence in their diagnosis even if their medical provider has rarely been confronted with the dynamics of this condition.

Research and Funding

Much research needs to be done to help establish the etiology, causes, and most effective treatment approaches for BBS. To date, anecdotal information has been the primary source of information in the pursuit of treatment and a cure BBS. We need to cull many more case histories before developing a working "grounded" hypothesis concerning the causes and onset of BBS. Studies need to be performed to attempt to quantify such issues as physical characteristics, family histories, environmental factors, and traumatic events to produce a body of evidence as to the complex, integrated causes.

To date, many possible explanations have been put forth for this condition, some eventually having been found to be without merit (such as the psychoanalytic perspective) and some consistent with the growing body of anecdotal evidence. The explanations, discussed throughout the book, have included cultural variables, toilet training, sexual abuse, homophobia, anxiety arousal caused by interpersonal space invasion, genetics, biochemical causes, obsessive-compulsive disorder, and psychoanalytic explanations such as the inability to express hostility, internalized wish for punishment, or "unconscious" association of urination with sexuality. Finally, it's important to recognize that urinary disease or prostate difficulties for men can cause difficulty with urination, and that such medical causes should be ruled out through an exam.

We need to begin thorough and rigorous multi-site studies to determine the most effective treatment approaches. There are a number of case studies and data from several anxiety disorder clinics across the country that strongly suggest what are effective and noneffective treatment strategies for paruretics.

For example, psychodynamic therapy, behavioral treatment, cognitive-behavioral treatment, paradoxical intention, hypnotherapy, and self-catheterization have all been reported to help in a limited number of cases. Still, there have been no controlled studies to date giving definitive evidence for the most effective treatment approaches. We do not know what method or methods, individually or combined, work best. Also, we do not know whether some methods work well for certain individuals (perhaps based on the etiology of the BBS), but not for others.

There is a vacuum of information as to which drugs, if any, are effective in the treatment of paruresis. There is anecdotal evidence that Cardura, Paxil, and Atenolol have worked for some individuals. But even here, it is not clear whether it was the drug itself or the drug in combination with some other form of treatment (e.g., graduated exposure therapy) that made the difference. Drug companies have not, as yet, addressed this specific question, though there are now treatments on the market for people with urinary frequency.

Finally, we don't know how long improvement lasts for treated clients. There is evidence from Himle's work that 40 percent keep their gains or improve, another 20 percent stay the same, and the final 40 percent report a partial or complete loss of gains previously made. Soifer's workshop data seems to indicate that most participants hold their gains after six months.

What is absolutely crucial at this juncture in the pursuit of defining, understanding, and treating paruresis is a carefully controlled study at three or four sites across the country. We would need at least forty to fifty paruretics at each site to participate in one of the following groups: a control group that was not administered treatment; a group that would receive supportive talk group treatment, but nothing else; a group that would receive behavior (graduated exposure) therapy; a group that would receive cognitive therapy; a group that would receive drug therapy; a group that would receive cognitive-behavioral therapy; a group that would receive drug and behavior therapy; a group that would receive drug and cognitive therapy; and a group that would receive drug and cognitive-behavioral therapy.

Until there is both a sufficient number of clients and funding to conduct such a massive study, we will not know for sure what the most effective treatment approaches are for BBS. Meanwhile, we will continue using the model that seems to hold the most promise—the graduated exposure approach. For those who suffer from paruresis and do not want to use this approach, we recommend that they talk to their physician about urinary self-catheterization, at least as an interim solution until further research can develop more effective treatments.

As one paruretic relates:

I'm a fifty-three-year-old married male, a professional scientist ... I've suffered with this problem since about eleven years of age. Traveling, especially plane travel, is extremely difficult for me and I've had to resort to such drastic measures as the use of indwelling catheters. (Not as horrendous as they sound.) I've derived a fair amount of solace from the knowledge that there are so many people whose minds are wired as mine—though I certainly wish there was some way to get the symptoms to leave each and everyone one of us.

Summary

Paruretics need to know that they are not alone. The chain of secrecy that keeps paruretics in a prison of isolation can only be broken through educating the general public, paruretics themselves, and, most importantly, health care providers about this problem and the havoc it wreaks on people who "coexist with the monkey." As interest is generated in the public through heightened awareness, funding for further research will naturally follow. Future research will yield crucial information that will lead to more effective treatment and the identification of causes that can trigger this condition. Thus, a two-pronged goal of treating this problem and educating the public will effectively address this devastating social phobia.

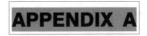

APPENDIX A

Literature Review

One of the most striking features of paruresis is the lack of attention it has received in the professional literature. With 17 million or more Americans experiencing some degree of difficulty when attempting to urinate in public rest rooms, such clinical inattention is dumbfounding. While we, the authors, could speculate endlessly as to why researchers have virtually ignored the topic, we instead present for those interested in more technical aspects, the following overview of the few reports available on bashful bladder syndrome (BBS). The early investigations into and reports on this subject primarily focused on the psychoanalytic approach—a model that has come under scrutiny in recent years. This information is provided in an attempt to be as thorough as possible regarding the evolution of the understanding of this syndrome.

Virtually all of the early reports on BBS focused exclusively on females, as well as on psychoanalytic and psychodynamic (Freudian) causes and treatments. For example, Wobus (1922) acknowledged the fact that urinary retention often occurred as a result of "emotional factors" rather than anatomical impairment. After reviewing the urological literature of the day, Pedersen (1923) found that only a few authors had cautiously referred to urinary retention as an hysterical reaction in some patients. Braasch and Thompson (1935) later confirmed the presence of a large number of women who complained of "urinary hesitancy" without any detectable organic causes, and suggested the presence of psychodynamic factors. Winsburg-White, et al. (1936) reported on two causes of urinary retention in women and used surgical resection of the bladder neck to successfully cure the patients. Menninger (1941) then discussed the significance of urination as an expression of sexual and aggressive impulses in Freudian terms. He proposed that urinary retention was an act of self-punishment for unacceptable sexual desires. Ritch (1946) suggested that urinary retention might best be treated by attending to the underlying psychological factors and conflicts generating the condition.

Emmett, Hutchins, and McDonald (1950) reported successfully treating 82 percent of their female patients who complained of urinary hesitancy by cutting a portion of the muscles of the urethral sphincters. In these cases the therapists noted a complete absence of organic disease or structural problems, and therefore suggested psychological causes. They also speculated that the disorder probably occurred more frequently than previously believed.

As part of the first comprehensive study of psychogenic urinary retention, in which they coined the term *paruresis*, Williams and Degenhardt (1954) administered a questionnaire containing the question: Do you find it difficult to pass urine in the presence of others? The authors found that at least 14 percent of the respondents reported urinary hesitancy. In addition, Williams and Degenhardt found a positive correlation between experiencing urinary hesitancy and experiencing discomfort when being watched at work, suggesting that paruretics are indeed social phobics.

Williams and Johnson (1956) described a woman who, as a child, had been physically, emotionally, and sexually abused by her aunt and uncle. The woman consequently focused her attention on genital and eliminative functions, and unconsciously confused urination with sexual activity. Because the woman experienced difficulty urinating whenever anger toward her relatives was about to surface, the therapists concluded that urinary retention symbolized the repression of hostile emotions.

Presenting a case study of a woman with BBS, Chapman (1959) reached similar conclusions. The patient, although not exposed to incest, experienced intense psychological stress as a result of murderous hostility toward her stepfather. Like Williams and Johnson's (1956) patient, the woman endured episodes of urinary retention whenever her rage was about to become conscious. Chapman also implied in this case that the localization of the symptom in the urinary system resulted from a childish desire to urinate on the mother's grave, as well as guilt associated with such an expression of hostility. After four years of psychodynamic therapy helped her to recognize and deal with her aggressive impulses, her urinary retention disappeared.

Knox (1960) speculated that a female patient developed paruresis following a transient episode of retention while giving birth. Knox also noted that the woman's resentment of pregnancy and desire to avoid further sexual intercourse served to maintain her symptoms. The woman's urinary retention ceased once she acknowledged and confronted her psychological issues.

Norden and Friedman (1961) presented a study of two women who experienced psychogenic urinary retention as a result of internalized conflicts. The therapists explained the first woman's inability to urinate as an attempt to cope with stress and repressed emotions. The second woman developed retention after hearing about the death of a friend from anuria (absence of urine production). Norden and Friedman indicated that both of these cases of urinary retention were psychosomatic and required long-term psychotherapy.

Scott, Quesada, and Cardus (1961) studied resistance to urinary flow in eleven healthy adult males. To accomplish this, the authors used a method that simultaneously measured sphincter action, bladder pressure, and urinary flow. They concluded that their method was a valuable means of determining the extent of hesitancy due to injury, drugs, and/or disease—the primary causes of urological difficulties in their sample.

Larson, Swenson, Utz, and Steinhilber (1963) studied thirty-seven female paruretics who ranged in age from thirteen to sixty-nine years. In the general absence of organic impairment in these patients, the therapists interviewed and administered several psychological tests. They found that the women tended to show hysterical personality characteristics, symptoms of depression and, in a few instances, schizophrenia. Many of the women spoke of various psychological problems and all voiced somatic complaints. Most of the patients related that a physically or emotionally stressful event had occurred prior to the onset of the urinary retention difficulty.

Wahl and Golden (1963) presented several case studies of individuals with BBS. Unlike studies conducted until that time, Wahl and Golden investigated both male and female patients with bladder retention problems. The therapists concluded that many diverse factors contributed to the development of paruresis in their patients. The first case presented concerned a woman whose urinary retention appeared to be due to sexual conflicts. According to the authors, because the woman's mother had warned her as a young woman to avoid sexual intercourse, urinary retention functioned as punishment for her promiscuity and as an indirect means to prevent sexual penetration. Next, the therapists investigated a woman who developed paruresis after disease sensitized her urinary system. In this case, problems in an unhappy marriage and an inability to express rage at an overly critical and unresponsive husband led to the localization of her urinary symptoms. Another case involved a male who unconsciously transferred fear and guilt onto his urinary functioning.

During psychotherapy the patient revealed the presence of a strong wish for the deaths of both his wife and mother, fear of death after witnessing a colleague die from urological disease, fear of being a homosexual, sexual excitement at witnessing the urine stream of other men, and several childhood fears regarding the size of his penis and masturbation.

Beginning in the mid-1960s, clinicians began using behavioral and other techniques, both with and without "talking" counseling, to treat BBS. Knowles (1964) described the case of an anxious female who had not previously responded to surgery, drug therapy, or psychotherapy. The therapist conducted seventeen sessions of hypnotherapy and reported that the woman was less tense and eventually was able to urinate easily several times each day. However, although her BBS improved, the woman continued to evidence other hysterical reactions, including swelling in her neck and losing her voice.

Margolis (1965) reviewed the available literature of the time. Noting that psychogenic urinary retention is both "a rather uncommon syndrome" and "not unusual," the author observed that the problem often arose following some form of social or psychological trauma, that the complainants were diagnosable as "neurotic or psychotic," and that no organic etiology was evident.

Cooper (1965) presented the case of a woman whose periodic episodes of BBS occurred in response to her relationship with a violent husband. The woman's retention led to several hospital admissions and served to remove her from a fearful home environment. The therapist, attempting to substitute an acceptable conditioned response for the psychogenic symptom, periodically injected the patient with carbachol (a parasympathetic stimulant) to induce involuntary episodes of diuresis. Later, the therapist substituted sterile water for the carbachol, and unexpectedly induced urination in the woman. The patient then responded to the sight of the syringe, and urinated at will. Thus Cooper, without the use of extensive counseling, treated BBS via a counterconditioning procedure. The therapist, however, cautioned that a change in the woman's marital situation was essential lest the newly counterconditioned response extinguish and the original urinary symptoms return.

Barnard, Flesher, and Steinbrook (1966), in treating a twenty-seven-year-old woman with BBS, speculated that "a sudden stress administered to an individual might induce a paradoxical rebound of the parasympathetic discharge." To that end, they seated the woman on a commode, applied electrodes to her legs, and ran a continuous electrical current until she voided. After several days of this therapy, the woman learned to administer the current herself and continued to urinate each time.

Using in vivo desensitization, Elliott (1967) treated a male paruretic who had obtained little symptomatic relief from traditional verbal counseling. During a series of twenty-eight sessions, the therapist moved progressively closer to the subject while he attempted to urinate in an isolated rest room. Eventually the patient was able to maintain a flow of urine when someone entered the lavatory, but continued to have difficulty initiating the process when someone else was already present. As part of a comprehensive behavioral program, Elliott provided counseling to teach the patient about "learning theory," as well as to help him to deal with his frustrations. Concerning future cases, the therapist stated that he would insist on more frequent sessions, use pleasurable behaviors (e.g., smoking) for purposes of reinforcement, and assure the patient that others suffer from the same condition. Elliott also admitted that his rigid adherence to learning principles while working almost exclusively with the patient's symptoms was responsible for the patient's limited success.

Tanagho and Miller (1970), in conducting dissection and tissue studies of the bladder as well as numerous studies into the mechanisms of micturition, concluded that no specific structure commonly termed the "internal urethral sphincter" exists. Instead, they proposed the presence of a "sphincter mechanism" including striated musculature around the urethral canal and the pelvic floor musculature—all of which function as a single system.

Khan (1971) presented a report of paruresis occurring in a young boy. The anxious nine-year-old entered the hospital after a two-day episode of acute retention. Repeated attempts at catheterization failed because of the extreme constriction of his urethral sphincters. Each episode of paruresis occurred whenever the boy encountered frustration, hostility, or anxiety that he was unable to handle. Once the patient participated in counseling, he recognized the relationship between his anger, anxiety, and inability to urinate.

Allen (1972) described six female paruretics who showed signs of internalized hostility. Interestingly, most of these women demonstrated schizoid and schizophrenic personality traits. The therapist concluded that urinary retention was an active expression of hostility and an acceptable substitute for venting anger. Stressing the importance of an accurate diagnosis, Allen noted that his paruretic patients responded well to psychological intervention.

Lamontagne and Marks (1973) treated two individuals, a male and a female, with BBS via a technique comparable to flooding a phobia. The therapists instructed the patients to drink considerable amounts of fluid before attending sessions, to enter the predetermined public lavatories, and then to produce urine, taking as long as they needed. As the treatment sessions continued, the therapists waited progressively closer to the rest rooms. The patients also practiced urinating while away from home, and ultimately voided in various public facilities without difficulty. Because both patients exhibited anxiety, shame, and nonassertiveness, the therapists concluded that BBS is a special type of social phobia. This being the case, the treatment appropriately required the patients to remain in the feared situation to reduce anxiety, no matter how painful. The therapists also suggested that avoidant behavior (leaving the public toilet before anxiety levels had lessened) had reinforced the maladaptive urinary symptoms.

Applying the principles of Davison's (1968) technique of orgasmic reorientation, Wilson (1973) treated a male paruretic who had not previously responded to systematic desensitization. Davison's procedure consisted of counterconditioning unacceptable sexual inclinations by linking conventional heterosexual stimuli to the stimulus of orgasm via a fading procedure. Using a similar method, Wilson directed the patient to continue voiding in familiar surroundings while visualizing someone entering the rest room at the moment when urination was certain. After two weeks, the patient was able to urinate comfortably while imagining someone standing next to him. Eventually the man was able to void easily in public facilities regardless of the number of individuals present.

Glasgow (1975) described a case report of a twenty-one-year-old male college student with BBS. The author used a fifteen-item anxiety hierarchy, systematic desensitization, and relaxation training. When this procedure failed, Glasgow had the patient drink large quantities of liquids and instituted a program of prolonged exposure, which eventually helped the patient urinate in various public facilities.

Ray and Morphy (1975) used systematic desensitization and metronome conditioned relaxation to treat a male with BBS. After reciting instructions for progressive relaxation above the soft beat of a metronome, the therapists presented fearful scenes from the patient's anxiety hierarchy. In addition, the man drank large quantities of fluids and was administered furosemide (a diuretic) before each session to improve the chances of successful voiding. The patient reported improvement after the fourth session, and discontinued therapy after the ninth session. Ray and Morphy noted that behavior therapy was the most effective means of treating phobias involving specific external objects and situations not related to internalized emotional factors.

Rees and Leach (1975), using questionnaires and interviews, found that between 25 percent and 50 percent of the 190 college males tested or interviewed reported periodically experiencing at least some degree of urinary hesitancy in public facilities. The authors determined the figure of 25 percent from responses to the question: "In a public rest room where someone is at the urinal (or in the stall) next to you, what are you most concerned about?" The possible answers included "noises," "odors," "size of penis," and "other (please specify)" with 25 percent of respondents choosing the "other" category and describing concern over initiating urination. Rees and Leach determined the figure 50 percent from the number of interviewees who expressed at least some anxiety over urinating in public facilities under certain conditions. As for BBS in women, Rees and Leach found that between 20 percent and 25 percent of 113 college females tested or interviewed reported experiencing occasional or chronic urinary hesitancy when using public rest rooms. Interesting, the authors found that males are more concerned than females about visual privacy in public rest rooms, while females are more concerned than males about auditory privacy.

Stanton (1976) concluded that urinary retention might be more common in women than had previously been suspected. In a review of fourteen cases, it was noted that, while some cases were due to bladder neck obstruction and inflammation, others (approximately 43 percent) had at least some concurrent psychological issue. Or, as the article put it, "Psychological problems, which were present in six of the fourteen cases, may possibly be relevant more often than in acute retention and may lead to the lax 'modesty' bladder, which is used to holding a large residue. Such cases, however, require detailed urodynamic and neurological assessment to exclude organic neurological disease" (1554).

Barrett (1976) studied psychogenic urinary retention in three women. Noting the need for a "combined approach" to treating cases of "psychogenic or hysterical retention of urine," the author recommended regular voidings, regulated fluid intake, intermittent catheterization, and psychiatric evaluation and treatment.

Middlemist, Knowles, and Matter (1976) proposed that the invasion of "personal space" was a critical factor in inhibiting urination. In their study, which involved secretly observing and measuring interpersonal distance at public urinals and urinary delay, the authors noted that certain cognitive states—tension, anxiety, and embarrassment—inhibited relaxation of the urethral sphincters. As a result, these cognitive states led certain individuals to experience urinary hesitancy, increased bladder pressure, and even acute retention. They commented that "the arousal model of personal space invasions proposes that close interpersonal distances are interpersonally stressful, increasing arousal and discomfort, and that it is this arousal that produces responses to invasions. . . . Both micturition delay and persistence were shown to be related to interpersonal distance" (545).

Anderson (1977) utilized in vivo systematic desensitization to treat five male paruretics. The patients devised and worked through anxiety hierarchies under the direction of the therapist. To enhance treatment, Anderson instructed the patients to wait until urinary urgency was great before entering a public lavatory, to approach more difficult situations only after anxiety in the easier situations had disappeared, and to remain in the rest room until either voiding occurred or three minutes had passed. The purpose of this three-minute requirement was to prevent reinforcing an avoidance response. Following therapy, each of the individuals reported being able to urinate at will in public rest rooms.

Employing the technique of paradoxical intention, Ascher (1979) treated five paruretics who had not previously responded to systematic desensitization, covert positive reinforcement, thought stopping, or in vivo assignments. The therapist instructed each of the patients to enter a busy lavatory whenever possible, to perform all of the activities associated with voiding, and to remain there for a reasonable length of time. Under no circumstances, however, were they to urinate. Once their performance anxiety diminished, the individuals typically broke the paradoxical directive and urinated. Subsequent therapy sessions emphasized the importance of inhibiting urination for as long as possible. Within six weeks, all of the patients reported reduced anxiety and the ability to urinate in public rest rooms with little or no difficulty. Consequently, Ascher affirmed the importance of paradoxical intention as an efficient means of dealing with the performance anxiety associated with BBS.

Montague and Jones (1979) treated five females and one male with BBS. The authors used a combination of biofeedback, relaxation training, guided imagery, psychotherapy, behavior therapy, drug therapy, and intermittent self-catheterization with generally good results. Christmas, Noble, Watson, and Turner-Warwick (1991) also used biofeedback to treat a young man with psychogenic urinary retention, and concluded that long-term behavioral therapies are the most effective intervention for this problem.

Weissberg and Levay (1979), based on their clinical experiences as psychiatrists, recommended that BBS be treated by exploring underlying psychodynamic conflicts and issues, such as concerns about penis size. The authors drew a similarity between BBS and sexual dysfunctions based on performance anxiety. They also noted that BBS is rarely seen as a presenting problem in mental therapy settings.

Bird (1980) reported on two cases of BBS in which analytic psychotherapy was used. In both patients, he noted a pattern of " unacceptable, unconscious sadistic and aggressive feelings," "intense desire for physical punishment [related to] guilt at repressed aggressive drives of considerable magnitude," as well as sensitivity to the invasion of personal body space. Thus, Bird proposed that intense and internalized anger, an inability to express emotions, guilt over hostile feelings, and an intense desire for punishment were significant factors in the development and maintenance of BBS. The author described sphincter disturbances as having an aggressive component, and urination as symbolizing the expression of hostility. Further, Bird noted that his patients were unable to project their anger onto others, and therefore resorted to psychogenic symptoms to punish themselves and others.

Palmtag and Reidasch (1980) performed "urodynamic analyses" on thirteen hundred patients, and found that of these only 2.7 percent experienced urinary difficulties due to psychogenic causes. Regarding urinary hesitancy in their sample, the authors found that urine retention was more typical of patients with psychoses, whereas a delay in flow was more typical of patients with psychosomatic disorders. They also concluded that it is possible to distinguish between psychogenic and neurogenic bladder problems with a neural sensitivity test.

Abramovici and Assael (1981) described three cases of BBS. The first involved a woman who periodically entered the hospital complaining of retention, but who consistently refused psychological intervention. Because of her husband's unfaithfulness, the woman resorted to urinary retention to receive attention, to avoid emotional issues, and to express sexual frustration through catheterizations. Next, Abramovici and Assael treated a mentally ill male paruretic. Emotional difficulties and the previous requirement of an indwelling catheter after a bladder injury appeared to be responsible for the development and localization of the psychosomatic symptom. The therapists final case concerned a woman who didn't recognize urinary urgency. Her denial of pain was consistent with repressed hostility toward her husband and their poor relationship. Thus, the therapists speculated that the woman's urinary retention and denial of accompanying pain were unconscious expressions of aggression and repulsion directed at her husband.

Gruber and Shupe (1982) administered a questionnaire to ninety male college students. They found that 32 percent reported "always," "usually," or "frequently" taking longer to initiate voiding with others present, compared to 68 percent who reported "occasionally," "seldom," or "never" having such difficulty. Gruber and Shupe also found a strong relationship between BBS and "body shyness," suggesting that paruretics are more likely to be bashful and reserved about their body and its functions.

Seif (1982) used hypnosis without the usual induction procedures to treat a male with BBS. After attempting a traditional induction, the therapist realized that the patient feared losing control during hypnotherapy. To alleviate the patient's anxiety, the therapist encouraged the patient instead to relax and think of a waterfall. After four sessions and several in vivo assignments, the man reported no further difficulty voiding in public facilities. Seif concluded that a nonthreatening and relaxed therapeutic environment was largely responsible for the patient's improvement. Mozdzierz (1985) also used hypnosis to treat a case of chronic urinary retention, though with the added strategy of paradoxical intention.

Stams, Martin, and Tan (1982) described the case of an eight-year-old boy with BBS. The therapists discovered through counseling that the youngster had come from an emotionally deprived and critical background. Also, the boy had previously injured his penis on a bicycle while being teased by some other children. The therapists speculated that the child developed BBS as a result of his fearing painful urination due to the earlier penile injury. A combination of drug therapy and induced motivation (e.g., offering the boy money for successful voiding) eventually eliminated the boy's urinary retention.

Jacob and Moore (1984) discussed the value of using paradoxical interventions to treat various behavioral disorders. Citing Ascher's (1979) work in this area, the authors explained:

> The acts of urination and defecation involve a complex interplay between behaviors that are under direct voluntary control (e.g., relaxation of external sphincters) and behaviors that are under autonomic nervous system control (e.g., relaxation of internal sphincters, contraction of the bladder detrusor muscle, contraction of colonic and rectal smooth muscle). . . . Trying too hard could paradoxically result in deterioration of the chain of behavior that leads to successful defecation or voiding. If patients respond to this deterioration by trying even harder, an exacerbation cycle is established for which paradoxical intention should be a viable treatment. (208)

Thyer and Curtis (1984) proposed that the duration of urination and the number of times that a patient successfully voided in public facilities were two important considerations when treating BBS via exposure therapy. To enhance urinary urgency, the therapists

122

administered furosemide to their patients one hour before the start of each therapy session. This procedure effected several voidings per hour, and thus facilitated the in vivo treatments. Unfortunately, the therapists didn't provide any further details about their patients or therapy methods.

In studying paruresis in the general population, Malouff and Lanyon (1985) described three forms of urinary retention: social inhibition involving momentary hesitancy; social inhibition involving inability to urinate in the presence of others with associated avoidant behavior and acute retention not related to social concerns. Malouff and Lanyon administered a questionnaire containing several scales to 381 college male subjects. They used the "avoidance" scale to determine the prevalence of BBS. Respondents reported how often they avoided campus rest rooms, bars, public events, and travel. Their findings suggested that about 7 percent of the general population suffers from "avoidant paruresis."

These same authors also used "inhibition," "introversion," "interpersonal anxiety," "performance anxiety," and "sexual anxiety" scales to gain further insights into BBS. Malouff and Lanyon found that the social cues most likely to trigger BBS included the presence and proximity of others in the rest room, absence of visual privacy, and the knowledge that someone else was waiting to use the facility. Avoidant paruretics also scored higher on scales measuring "interpersonal anxiety" and "performance anxiety."

Kawabe and Niijima (1987) used an alpha-1-blocker to treat five women with "micturition difficulties of unknown origin." The author's concluded that alpha blockers, which have also been used to treat enlarged prostates, may be useful for treating mild cases of urinary difficulty.

MacCaulay, Stern, Holmes, and Stanton (1987) administered questionnaires to assess the mental status of 211 women seeking services from a urological clinic. Those with urinary difficulties tended to exhibit psychiatric symptoms of anxiety, phobias, and depression. The authors also found that the urinary symptoms of about one-fourth of the women studied created an "intolerable" life situation for them.

Zgourides (1987) reviewed the literature to date on paruresis, and also recommended that a multidimensional treatment program—including such techniques as in vivo desensitization, paradoxical intention, rational-emotive, and cognitive therapies—would probably prove helpful in at least some cases. Moreover, Zgourides (1988) suggested using parasympathomimetic compounds such as bethanechol chloride (to induce voiding) as a possible adjunct to psychological exposure therapies.

Bassi, Zattoni, Aragona, Dal Bianoc, Calabro, and Artibani (1988) proposed that psychogenic urinary retention is a rare event. In their examination of six cases, the authors noted that, in the absence of physiological obstruction, psychic trauma can and does play a role in inhibiting the start of urination—leading to a diagnosis of psychogenic urinary retention.

Kitami, Masuda, Chiba, and Kumagai (1989) reported on two cases of psychogenic urinary retention—one female and one male. Cystometry showed that both subjects had "hypoactive bladders" with no evidence of detrusor sphincter dysfunction. Both were treated with a combination of counseling, intermittent self-catheterization, diazepam, and bethanechol.

In treating two cases of BBS, one male and one female, Zgourides, Warren, and Englert (1990) used a portable radio headset as an adjunct to in vivo therapy. Both paruretics became extremely anxious at the thought of someone hearing them urinate. In separate therapy sessions, both patients voided almost immediately when the therapists wore the headset. This was in sharp contrast to the usual significant delays the patients experienced in initiating voiding.

Hatterer, Gorman, Fyer, and associates (1990) treated four males who had BBS with a selective beta-blocker (atenolol) and/or a MAO inhibitor (phenelzine). All of the patients experienced uncomfortable side effects and only one reported improvement with atenolol.

Zgourides and Warren (1990) administered a beta-blocker (propranolol) to a male paruretic in the hopes of decreasing contraction of his urethral sphincters. Although the drug therapy did nothing to decrease his urinary symptoms, the patient reported a decrease in other autonomic symptoms (e.g., tachycardia) that at times had worsened his urinary difficulties in public rest rooms. Similarly, Zgourides (1991) attempted the use of the beta-blocker atenolol with another male paruretic. The results were essentially the same as in the previous case; the patient experienced no relief from his urinary symptoms.

McCracken and Larkin (1991) used in vivo desensitization and relaxation training to treat a thirty-seven-year-old male who had had BBS since the age of twelve. Treatment followed a standard protocol of graduated exposure over a series of twenty-three sessions, after which the patient expressed confidence in his ability to urinate for a drug screening.

Nicolau, Toro, and Prado (1991) treated a thirteen-year-old girl with a progressively worsening case of paruresis who spent as many as twelve hours each day urinating. The authors used a combination of family therapy, cognitive restructuring, and systematic desensitization to reduce the girl's maladaptive urinary behaviors and intense fear of urinating.

Markway, Carmin, Pollard, and Flynn (1992) described two individuals with BBS. "Amy" reported anxiety at the thought of using busy airport rest rooms, where she believed other women who were in line to use the toilet were thinking "Why is she taking so long?" and "What could she possibly be doing in there?" "Dave" reported anxiety at the possibility of not being to urinate right away. He worried along the lines of "What if the other men think I'm some kind of pervert?" and "They might think I'm masturbating because I'm taking so long," and "What if they think I'm gay?" For these individuals and other paruretics, Markway et al. recommended a combination of exposure, relaxation training, and cognitive restructuring.

Caffaratti, Perez-Rodriguez, Garat, and Farre (1993) studied an acute case of psychogenic urinary retention in a young female child. The authors concluded that, while acute psychogenic urinary retention is not common in adults, it is even less common in children.

Willimon (1994) reported in an issue of *USA Today* magazine on Himle's exposure method, which requires between six and ten weekly hour-long sessions. Patients arrive for sessions with a full bladder, and then confront a variety of rest rooms as they gradually work up to more crowded, "difficult" public facilities. The program involves cognitive restructuring and gradual desensitization to public rest rooms.

Bosio, Mazzucchelli, and Sandri (1996) explained that some young children experience urinary retention due to psychogenic causes. They also recommended that the earlier childhood urinary problems can be treated, the better. The authors described the case of a three-year-old boy with both urinary and fecal retention who responded favorably over a period of five years to a combination of interventions involving assorted clinicians, psychologists, teachers, social workers, and educators.

Zgourides (1996) developed a method of managing BBS via clean, intermittent self-catheterization. The therapist suggested this procedure to a male paruretic who had a long history of failed therapeutic attempts to treat his urinary condition. Following extensive consultation with a urologist, and after Zgourides and the patient created a portable "catheter pack," the man reported using this sure fire method whenever the need to urinate reached emergency levels.

Bohn and Sternbach (1997) briefly highlighted the research published to date on paruresis. They noted that the professional literature is lacking in the areas of prevalence of the disorder, etiology, controlled experimentation, pharmacological interventions, and psychological methods. As the authors noted, there exists a ". . . current lack of knowledge regarding the relationship of paruresis with psychiatric disorders in general ... [and] the need for conducting drug therapy research of paruresis in patients with social phobia and other anxiety disorders" (42).

An article in the Malegrams section of the October 1997 issue of *Men's Health* suggested that male paruretics loosen up by the following three methods. The author recommended visualizing relaxing things and a running faucet, not worrying about the amount of time it takes to start urinating, and using a stall instead of a urinal.

Labbate (1997) examined the issue of urine drug testing of paruretics. The nature of paruresis makes it impossible for those with severe cases to produce urine on cue for employers, the military, etc., even after extended periods of trying. Labbate concluded that while not a rare event, paruresis seems difficult to treat particularly by strictly pharmacological means" (250).

Goodwin, Swinn, and Fowler (1998) studied women with urinary retention, and recommended neuromodulation as an intervention. This method involves the "insertion of the percutaneous nerve evaluation (PNE) lead," which in turn produces "spectacular" results (305).

Jaspers (1998) reported the successful treatment of a sixteen-year-old male paruretic via cognitive restructuring and gradual in vivo exposure. The author concluded that while a multidimensional approach to treating BBS is desirable, clinicians should pay more attention to the cognitive components of the disorder. Jaspers also noted that using medications to treat BBS holds little promise.

Kroll, Martynski, and Jankowski (1998) used the phrase "lazy bladder syndrome" to describe a case of psychogenic urinary retention. The authors wrote of a fourteen-year-old girl admitted to a local hospital with an episode of urinary retention of twenty hours duration. Treatment included intermittent catheterization, alpha-blockade, and psychotropic medications. Kroll, Martynski, and Jankowski recommended that both biological and psychological factors be considered in cases of "lazy bladder syndrome."

Van der Linden and Venema (1998) explained that acute urinary is rather uncommon, affecting only 0.07 per one thousand Dutch citizens each year. Besides gynecological tumors being the most common obstructive cause of urinary retention, psychogenic factors can play a role. The authors contended that the diagnosis of psychogenic urinary retention must only be made when all other causes have been excluded.

Fukui, Nukui, Kontani, Nagata, Kurokawa, Katsuta, Sugimura, Okamoto, and Komatsu (1999) studied twenty-two patients with psychogenic urinary retention as part of a larger study on psychogenic lower urinary tract infections in women. Through psychological testing and interviews, they found the presence of subconscious defense mechanisms and suppression, which affected urinary ability. The authors concluded that an accurate diagnosis of psychogenic urinary retention requires a variety of psychological, anatomical, and traditional urological tests.

Rosario, Chapple, Tophill, and Woo (2000) studied forty men with bashful bladders who were unable to urinate during routine urodynamic testing (i.e., video cystometrography). The subjects were males with a median age of 51.9 years and various urological complaints. After attaching portable electronic recorders and allowing the men to urinate in private, the researchers concluded that the bashful bladder syndrome was not related to any specific urological diagnosis. They also found surgery to be helpful in 20 percent of men over forty.

Final Comments

As is readily apparent from the above case summaries, psychotherapists have utilized a number of techniques to treat BBS. Yet none alone has proven to be universally effective. Therefore, because the etiologies and degree of affliction vary so much among individuals, a multidimensional approach to the condition would seem to be the most reasonable.

What is the best overall treatment for BBS? The authors collectively believe, based on literature, anecdotal evidence, and clinical experience, that an individualized approach is necessary to maximize success for the BBS patient. A multidimensional approach including talking therapy, graduated exposure and desensitization therapy, and (when indicated) drug therapy, combines the most effective treatments and affords the patient the greatest opportunity to overcome this social phobia.

Evolution of the Bathroom, and Its Impact on Paruresis

How modern man (and woman) deal with the problem of human elimination has shown much variation across time, civilizations, and religions. The only reason it would even appear to be an issue is because we are social beings, and are concerned about how and what others think of us. Living in groups, the individual, to some degree, must conform to group norms in order to maintain his or her position within the group (Kira 1970, 1976).

Moreover, the affluence of a society will shape the kinds of facilities that eventually develop. Initially, one would expect some collective facility, then perhaps several smaller facilities for subgroups or families, and finally individual toilet facilities in private dwellings. A key factor would also be the availability of water for disposal purposes (Kira 1976).

Early in the human species' evolution, bathrooms were clearly unnecessary, since we wandered about without any permanent settlements, and used the outdoors and earth to relieve ourselves and cover our excrement. Once we established some roots, however, and built dwellings, the need for facilities for the disposal of human bodily waste was necessary. Consequently, primitive toilets were created, first outside of any dwelling units, and then eventually moved indoors. Of course, just moving these early toilet facilities indoors wasn't enough, since the odors could become overwhelming with time. So various methods were developed to deal with the situation (Pathak 1995).

Rome pioneered the men's public urinal, which was referred to as the "pissoir" or "Vespasienne." Either simply out in the open or with a minimal degree of privacy, these devices collected the urine for the use as dye, which was sold by Emperor Vespasian to fatten his coffers (Kira 1976). They were also a means to try to prevent the commoner from simply urinating in the stairwells of buildings (Horan 1997).

As incredible as it may seem, almost a thousand years passed between the fall of the Roman Empire and the restoration of public (and to a large degree, private) toilets in Europe, though Constantinople continued the Roman tradition of public sewage disposal (Newman 1997).

The year 1596 C.E. was a watershed; the Englishman J. D. Harrington invented the water closet, or WC (Pathak 1995). Of course, this was merely an improvement on an ancient design (the Palace of Knossos), the key difference being that the WC had moving parts. The WC, or toilet as we know it in the United States, was placed in a small room somewhere in the home. While its introduction was initially shunned by decent people, today it would be hard to imagine living without it, some saying it "marks man's final ascent to civilization" (Horan 1997, 204). Believe it or not, it took a full 200 years before the WC became popular during the late 1700s. In the 1850s, Thomas Crapper, another Englishman, had the distinction of developing the toilet design that is still used today (Horan 1997).

In 1739, a Parisian restaurant, for the first time, provided separate facilities for the different sexes at a dance. In 1824, the first public toilet facilities appeared in France (Pathak 1995). This may seem remarkable, but it highlights a very important point. The whole idea of "privacy" in using the toilet is a very modern concept, with its origins in the 1800s (Newman 1997). It is important to remember that the notion of "personal privacy" has evolved over the last couple of hundred years, and is tied to both economic prosperity and religious notions. As one observer has aptly stated: "One obviously has to have the conditions that permit modesty before a society can make modesty into an operable virtue" (Kira 1976, 6). What might seem incredible to us moderns today are probably pre-Enlightenment (and certainly pre-Victorian!) attitudes toward elimination.

Prior to the twentieth century, only the well-to-do had WC, or flush, toilets. The other classes had to make due with outdoor privies or "earth closets" (wooden seat and pail below) in a small room or in furniture, often referred to as a "potty chair." Elaborate effort went into disguising these devices (Newman 1997, 92–93).

The middle classes, especially in the cities, began to have toilets installed in their homes en masse beginning in the late 1800s and early 1900s. Functionality, not design, was the hallmark of the day (Kira 1976). It's important to realize that another factor preventing mass installation of toilets, either personal or public ones, was the lack of sewage treatment, which did not develop until 1889 (Pathak 1995). Prior to this, despite the fact that the Romans had developed underground sewers many centuries ago, most sewage was disposed of in open gutters lining city streets.

As we have seen, the history of public toilets is pretty scanty. In some parts of the world, people still do their business wherever they are, whenever they want to. The two key factors influencing our habits have been public health concerns and the rise of large cities. Kira (1976) defines the public toilet as "one that is provided in the interest of public convenience, sanitation, and health in a communal location by, or on behalf of, a communal agency for use by anyone with need" (193–94).

Why do people even need public facilities in the first place? One reason, of course, is not having access to a private bathroom (which in the case of today's homeless population is not uncommon at all). But we all occasionally need public toilets, that is, when we're not at home and are "caught short" either at work, socializing, or traveling. Both scenarios have influenced the design of public toilets (Kira 1976).

Once again, Paris led the way with the reintroduction of men's public urinals in the 1840s, the first since Roman Emperor Vespasian's time! Many, like in Roman times, were wide open; only some offered any privacy. The French also pioneered "fully enclosed kiosks" for women beginning in the 1860s. In the 1880s, water closets began to appear, which could be used by either gender. With rail travel came the impetus to build public rest rooms to accommodate passengers in the terminals, marking the real advent of such facilities (Kira 1976).

Met with initial skepticism, by the end of the nineteenth century, public rest rooms were an accepted fact in the large cities of Europe and the United States. Initially clean and friendly, they have tended to deteriorate over the years. As commercial and retail businesses developed in the twentieth century, and building codes required them to have bathrooms for their customers, municipalities no longer felt required to provide them. Moreover, along with new forms of transportation, the subway, car, and airplane, came new forms of public (and private) restroom facilities. Finally, the growth of the state and federal park system, as well as the popularity of camping, raised issues of rest room design for the so-called "wilderness" (Kira 1976, 196).

The introduction of automobiles led to the rise of gas stations across the country. No longer able to simply get by with outdoor privies in the back, they needed to provide toilets for men and women. Also, as the federal interstate system developed, so did the need for public facilities along the highways. Finally, all of this travel by car helped the hotel and motel industry, too, which also had to build toilets for travelers (Kira 1976).

In thinking about the above history, it is important to understand current attitudes toward "territoriality and privacy." While many, if not most, of us have positive or at least neutral feelings toward the bathrooms in our apartment or houses, when it comes to public rest rooms, many of us have negative feelings toward them. This often has to do with their layout and/or how well they are or are not maintained. Says Kira (1976):

> Most of our feelings about the body, sex, elimination, privacy, and cleanliness are magnified in this context of "publicness," for the fact of publicness, with its inevitable territorial violations and lost of privacy, increases our apprehensions (200).

According to an IKEA (the home furnishing store) survey, the number-one reason people work at home is "to avoid having to use a communal bathroom" (PR Newswire, 2000).

It is possible that we project this negativity onto what we find in public facilities, including the urinals, toilets, and perhaps even the strangers in there. If we fear the stranger, and suspect that our personal space may be violated, then the situation will not be conducive to our doing our business there, whether it is urination or defecation. And, even if we are neutral about our own bodily eliminations, we are certainly less so about others, especially if we see what is essentially supposed to be private or unseen (Kira 1976).

The well-known sociologist Erving Goffman speaks of "territories of the self," which relates to what is perceived to be mine, in this case, in relation to personal space. If we have to create a temporary space that we perceive as ours in what is essentially a public facility, and this space becomes violated in some way, then we are likely to have a psychological reaction to it (Kira 1976, 201–02). In some cases, we would argue, this reaction is paruresis.

Two key ideas here are "privacy-from" and "privacy-for." The former arises most often in public facilities. We don't want to be around others doing their business. So it becomes essential to protect ourselves from them. Again, Goffman is helpful here; he speaks of "civil inattention" as a way to create such protection. Says Kira (1976):

> This device of scrupulously observed avoidance behavior
> is widely employed in many cultures and situations and

demands that we avoid observing other people's behavior and in particular . . . that we avoid making eye contact. (201–02)

Thus, in a public rest room, etiquette requires that men not make eye contact and certainly do not look at each other's private parts. Also, spacing at urinals becomes an issue; for example, if there are three next to each other, and someone is at one end, the next person will go to the other end. Only if there isn't a free urinal will we go next to someone else. Otherwise, it may raise suspicions. Several exceptions exist to this general rule, in particular school and the military, institutions that attempt to enforce conformity by getting rid of privacy (Kira 1976).

"Privacy-for" is one of the guiding principles of home bathroom design. When extended to the public facilities design, the following concerns become important: "a discreet location; discreet identification; the use of visual barriers or compartments; [and] the use of masking sounds, most commonly piped in music" (Kira 1976, 205). Interestingly, there is much variation in this regard from culture to culture, especially in the area of visual protection. For example, European water closets are completely enclosed, affording maximum privacy to their temporary guests. In the United States, the standard design for stalls are sides and a door that start one foot above the floor and extend only five and a half feet in total height (Kira 1976). It is our observation that while Europeans, in general, detest U.S. public restroom designs, U.S. travelers abroad, especially paruretics, are often delighted with European standards and consider them more "civilized."

While social convention dictates that most people will generally ignore others in public rest rooms, this is not very comforting to paruretics. Many simply avoid going in public at all costs. Women who do so are prone to get into physical trouble; according to Kira (1976), holding their urine was the cause of bladder infections for over half of the women in several studies. For the other gender, Kira (1976) notes:

> Lack of privacy, or more particularly, lack of privacy to the degree demanded by any given individual, can have unfortunate consequences. The most serious . . . is usually its inhibiting effect on elimination function, most often male urination. . . . Although it may strike some as surprising that this is still a problem . . . the advice columns of the newspapers carry letters asking about these problems with great regularity (206–07).

As if all of what we have discussed so far wasn't enough, there are other factors that affect people's attitudes toward urination and defecation. For some, there may be a conscious or unconscious association of these activities, primarily urination, with sex, since the same organ, at least visibly, serves two functions. Moreover, there may be deep seated "moral taboos" about keeping our genitals covered and not touching them in public, both of which are violated in public rest room situations. Finally, it seems that both men and women generally experience discomfort in making noise while eliminating, especially if others are around to hear them (Kira 1976).

There appear to be huge differences between cultures in elimination positions, especially regarding urination. What we found most startling is that the respective urination positions for men and women that we take for granted in modern society appear to have been reversed in the past! For example, Herodotus claimed that in Egypt, "women stand erect to make water, the men stoop"; in Ireland, "the men discharge their urine sitting; the women standing"; among Muslims, both genders "squat to defecate and urinate." And European women, until quite recently, would often stand up to urinate, as their clothing almost dictated that position, and they could do so quite discreetly. Finally, many women today, because of the lack of cleanliness in public facilities, will not sit on the toilet seat to urinate, and instead either hover or stand up. Lest anyone think that men, at least in Western society, feel comfortable sitting down to urinate, all we have to do is recall that when President Lyndon Johnson heard that someone in his Administration was dovish on the Vietnam war, he reputedly said: "Hell, he has to squat to piss!" (Kira 1976, 104–05)

We can now better understand how certain issues come together for paruretics. As Kira (1976) comments:

> Since the entire sex-elimination amalgam is something we tend to think of as "dirty" and something to be somewhat ashamed of, we also tend to want to hide and disguise our involvement with it; in other words, we seek privacy for it ... [and] we resort to all sorts of stratagems to avoid anyone's knowing where we are or what we are about (107).

The desire for modesty and some degree of privacy seem normal when it comes to something as private as personal elimination. While Kira (1976) feels that this desire, if taken to the extreme (that is, wanting complete privacy), can create a problem in that people may not be able to eliminate without these cues, from our point of view what is viewed as normal or not normal is far from clear. For example, Kira (1976) states that many have difficulty providing urine samples in a doctor's office without sufficient privacy. At least one urologist has told us that one-third of his patients cannot provide a urine sample on demand. So, what is the problem? Clearly, insufficient privacy. Furthermore, even Kira (1976) says that one survey indicates that more than half of us will stop either temporarily or for the duration of our elimination activities if someone else is in too close proximity either at home or in a public rest room.

The need for privacy, then, seems to be important to many men and women when it comes to elimination functions. According to Kira (1976), at least three levels of privacy can be discerned:

> 1) privacy of being heard, but not seen, 2) privacy of not being seen or heard, and 3) privacy of not being seen, heard, or sensed—in other words, other people should not even be aware of one's whereabouts or action. It is probably fair to say, however, that these categories generally represent degrees of tolerable privacy rather than degrees of desired privacy, in the sense that, given a choice, most people would, for these purposes, tend to pick maximum privacy. The degree of tolerable privacy varies enormously, depending on the activity and the particular individual. (165)

It would seem that those who are most "negative or apprehensive" about "disgusting things" like elimination would have the most difficulty with others around, and thereby require the most privacy for it (Kira 1976, 164). While this may be a psychological fact for some, it seems that several other factors, both social and environmental, come into play, too. Interestingly, the home bathroom is the only "off-bounds" space in most homes, and thus the only place people can have total privacy for whatever needs (positive or negative) they have. The privacy afforded by the bathroom at home serves another function: reducing our shame and embarrassment while engaged in a private activity. While this may be a current "cultural norm" (recall that even in the recent past privacy for anything, including elimination, was virtually non-existent), it is almost universally accepted today (Kira 1976).

The puritanical roots of our Anglo-Saxon culture may partially explain our fastidiousness around not only privacy in the bathroom, but gender-specific public toilets. One can see how strongly this runs by observing people's behavior around single-stall locked bathrooms: virtually no one will use an opposite gender toilet even if it is empty and there is a line for your own gendered one. It seems that for a period of time in the liberal 1960s and early 1970s, several countries, such as England, France, Italy, and Japan, had no such compunctions, and unisex public facilities were commonplace. This may still be somewhat true today, but our impression is that many countries are moving toward the more conservative moral (and political) standards of the United States.

Public rest rooms in many places leave something to be desired. Many, it seems, provide "unbelievably minimal, cramped, and filthy facilities." One survey of over 500 facilities in New York City in the early 1970s showed that about 70 percent of them had something wrong with them. And an American Automobile Association (AAA) survey around the same time indicated that "dirty rest rooms" came in second on the complaint list (Kira 1976, 212–14).

How are public rest rooms in various establishments, whether bars, restaurants, train stations, interstate rest areas, or airports, designed and built? What governs the number of urinals and toilets that are installed in these facilities?

Various building codes—either state, county, or city—guide the number of urinals and toilet fixtures in any particular building. These codes, however, only minimally address design issues, and usually only regulate things such as spacing and height. The Americans with Disabilities Act (ADA) also governs the number of handicapped accessible urinals and toilets that must be installed.

When a particular establishment puts out bids to construction firms for a contract, the primary concern at both ends that governs the design of rest rooms is cost. Those paying to have public rest rooms built want to minimize costs, and those bidding on a potential contract will put in the lowest bid possible. Consequently, architects designing the plans will try and recommend the least expensive alternatives that will meet minimum code requirements. This leads to several problems.

Men, even those who aren't paruretic, face several problems when it comes to elimination in a public urinal. Least among these is back splash; however, this problem is compounded when there are no dividers, and men hug the urinal to afford some form of privacy. Also, urinals are often spaced so close together that in a crowded situation, one is virtually touching the next person's elbows. It's estimated that at least another foot of space is needed between urinals in many men's rooms. Kira (1976, 230) states that "from the standpoint of privacy and of clearly defining the 'territory' of each urinal, it would be desirable if dividers were incorporated between fixtures." We would go much further than that. We would argue that all urinals must have dividers between them, preferably floor to ceiling ones that mostly or completely block out the sight of the person standing next to you. Moreover, low-bowl urinals should be discontinued.

For women, the problems are different. Since it appears that the "vast majority" of women don't sit on the toilet seat anyway (fully 96 percent in a 1970s British survey), it would seem that a redesign of women's toilets is in order. The basic concern is getting venereal disease, which can happen. There are several innovative designs that would allow women to be in the more comfortable "semi-sitting" or "hovering" position (Kira 1976, 232–37).

One solution we would propose for both men's and women's public rest rooms, particularly for paruretics, is having at least several fully enclosed water closets installed in every public facility, as is the custom in most European countries. This would afford almost complete privacy for the user, and go a long way toward helping paruretics overcome their avoidance of public rest rooms.

For Further Help

If you're interested in learning more about bashful bladder syndrome, attending a workshop, or finding out how you can become involved in disseminating information, you're invited to contact: Steven Soifer, M.S.W., Ph.D., President; The International Paruresis Association, Inc. (IPA, Inc.); P.O. Box 26225; Baltimore, Maryland 21210. Phone: 1-800-247-3864; fax: 1-410-706-6046.

Dr. Soifer works with individual clients, conducts day-long or weekend workshops, and helps set up support groups throughout the world.

For those of you with Internet access, the paruresis website address is: http://www.paruresis.org or http://www.shybladder.org.

Psychologists Joseph Himle, M.S.W., Ph.D., and George Zgourides, Psy.D., see patients with parureticin their private practices. Dr. Himle may be reached at: University of Michigan Medical Center; Anxiety Disorders Program; 1500 E. Medical Center Drive, Room C435; Ann Arbor, MI 48109-0840. Phone: 734-426-5684.

Dr. Zgourides, who works with paruresis clients over the phone and in-person, may be reached at: www.CounselorsOnCall.com or georgezgourides@juno.com.

References

Abramovici, I., and M. Assael. 1981. Psychogenic retention of urine. *Psychiatria Clinica* 14:196-204.

Allen, T. D. 1972. Psychogenic urinary retention. *Southern Medical Journal* 65:302-304.

American Psychiatric Association. 1994. *The Diagnostic and Statistical Manual of Mental Disorders.* 4th ed. Washington, D.C.: APA.

Anderson, L. T. 1977. Desensitization in vivo for men unable to urinate in a public facility. *Journal of Behavior Therapy and Experimental Psychology* 8:105-106.

Ascher, L. M. 1979. Paradoxical intention in the treatment of urinary retention. *Behaviour Research and Therapy* 17:267-270.

Barnard, G., C. Flesher, and R. Steinbrook. 1966. The treatment of urinary retention by aversive stimulus cessation and assertive training. *Behaviour Research and Therapy* 4:231-236.

Barrett, D. M. 1976. Psychogenic urinary retention in women. *Mayo Clinic Proceedings* 51:351-356.

Bassi, P., F. Zattoni, F. Aragona, M. Dal Bianco, A. Calabro, and W. Artibani. 1988. Psychogenic urinary retention of urine in women: Diagnostic and therapeutic problems. *Journal of Urology Paris* 94:159-162.

Bird, J. R. 1980. Psychogenic urinary retention. *Psychotherapy and Psychosomatics* 34:45-51.

Bohn, P., and H. Sternbach. 1997. Current knowledge and research directions in the treatment of paruresis. *Depression and Anxiety* 5:41-42.

Bosio, M., S. Mazzucchelli, and S. Sandri. 1996. Psychogenic urinary retention in childhood: A severe case treated by an integrated global approach. *Minerva Pediatrician* 48:117-120.

Bourne, E. J. 1998. *Healing Fear: New Approaches to Overcoming Anxiety.* Oakland, Calif.: New Harbinger.

————. 1995. *The Anxiety and Phobia Workbook.* 2nd ed. Oakland, Calif.: New Harbinger.

Braasch, W. F., and G. J. Thompson. 1935. Treatment of the atonic bladder. *Surgery, Gynecology and Obstetrics* 61:379-384.

Caffaratti, J., S. Perez-Rodriguez, J. M. Garat, and L. Farre. 1993. Acute urinary retention of psychogenic cause in a girl. *Actas Urology Espanola* 17:367-370.

Chapman, A. H. 1959. Psychogenic urinary retention in women: Report of a case. *Psychosomatic Medicine* 21: 119-122.

Christmas, T. J., J. G. Noble, G. M. Watson, and R. T. Turner-Warwick. 1991. Use of biofeedback in treatment of psychogenic voiding dysfunction. *Urology* 37:43-45.

Cooper, A. J. 1965. Conditioning therapy in hysterical retention of urine. *British Journal of Psychiatry* 111:575-577.

Davis, M., E. R. Eshelman, and M. McKay. 1995. *The Relaxation and Stress Reduction Workbook.* 4th ed. Oakland, Calif.: New Harbinger.

Davison, G. C. 1968. Elimination of a sadistic fantasy by a client-controlled counter-conditioning technique: A case study. *Journal of Abnormal Psychology* 73:84-90

Elliott, R. 1967. A case of inhibition of micturition: unsystematic desensitization. *Psychological Record* 17:525-530.

Ellis, A. 1962. *Reason and Emotion in Psychotherapy.* New York: Lyle Stuart.

Emmett, J. L., S. P. R. Hutchins, and J. R. McDonald. 1950. The treatment of urinary retention in women by transurethral resection. *Journal of Urology* 63:1031-1042.

Fezler, W. 1989. *Creative Imagery: How to Visualize in All Five Senses.* New York: Simon and Schuster.

Fukui, J., F. Nukui, K. Kontani, M. Nagata, J. Kurokawa, M. Katsuta, T. Sugimura, S. Okamoto, and H. Komatsu. 1999. Psychogenic lower urinary tract dysfunction in women: Pathophysiological investigation for psychogenic frequency-urgency syndrome and psychogenic urinary retention. *Nippon Hinykika Gakkai Zasshi* 90:769-778.

Glasgow, R. E. 1975. In vivo exposure in the treatment of urinary retention. *Behavior Therapy* 6:701-702.

Goodwin, R. J., M. J. Swinn, and C. J. Fowler. 1998. The neurophysiology of urinary retention in young women and its treatment by neuromodulation. *World Journal of Urology* 16:305-307.

Gruber, D. L, and D. R. Shupe. 1982. Personality correlates of urinary hesitancy paruresis and body shyness in male college students. *Journal of College Student Personnel* 23:308-313.

Hatterer, J. A., J. M. Gorman, A. J. Fyer, R. Campeas, F. R. Schneier, E. Hollander, L. A. Papp, and M. R. Liebowitz. 1990. Clinical and research reports: Pharmacotherapy for four men with paruresis. *American Journal of Psychiatry* 147:109-111.

Horan, J. L. 1997. *The Porcelain God: A Social History of the Toilet.* Secaucus: Citadel Press.

Jacob, R. G., and D. J. Moore. 1984. Paradoxical interventions in behavioral medicine. *Journal of Behavior Therapy and Experimental Psychiatry* 15:205-213.

Jaspers, J. P. 1998. Cognitive-behavioral therapy for paruresis: A case report. *Psychological Reports* 83:187-196.

Johnson, S. L. 1997. *Therapist's Guide to Clinical Intervention.* San Diego, Calif.: Academic Press.

Kawabe, K., and T. Niijima. 1987. Use of an alpha1-blocker, YM-12617, in micturition difficulty. *Urology International* 42:280-284.

Kessler, R. C., M. B. Stein, and P. Berglund. 1997. *Social Phobia Subtypes in the National Co-Morbidity Study.* Boston: Department of Health Care Policy, Harvard Medical School.

Khan, A. U. 1971. Psychogenic urinary retention in a boy. *Journal of Urology* 106:432-434.

Kira, A. 1970. Privacy in the bathroom. In *Environmental Psychology: Man and his Physical Setting,* edited by H. M. Proshansky, W. H. Ittelson, and L. B. Rivlin. New York: Holt, Rinehart and Winston.

———. 1976. *The Bathroom.* New York: Viking.

Kitami, K., M. Masuda, K. Chiba, and H. Kumagai. 1989. Psychogenic urinary retention: Report of two cases. *Hinyokika Kiyo* 35:509-512.

Knowles, F. W. 1964. Hypnotherapy in chronic hysterical urinary retention: Report of a case. *New Zealand Medical Journal* 63:38-40.

Knox, S. J. 1960. Psychogenic urinary retention after parturition, resulting in hydronephrosis. *British Medical Journal* 2:1422-1424.

Kroll, P., M. Martynski, and A. Jankowski. 1998. The role of psychogenic factors as a cause of urinary retention in a patient with lazy bladder syndrome. *Wiad Lek* 51: 102-5.

Kurtz, L. F. 1997. *Self-Help and Support Groups: A Handbook for Practitioners*. Thousand Oaks, Calif.: Sage.

Labbate, L. A. 1997. Paruresis and urine drug testing. *Depression and Anxiety* 4:249-252.

Lamontagne, Y., and I. M. Marks. 1973. Psychogenic urinary retention: Treatment by prolonged exposure. *Behavior Therapy* 4:581-585.

Larson, J. W., W. M. Swenson, D. C. Utz, and R. M. Steinhilber. 1963. Psychogenic urinary retention in women. *Journal of the American Medical Association* 184:697-700.

Macaulay, A. J., R. S. Stern, D. M. Holmes, and S. Stanton. 1987. Micturition and the mind: Psychological factors in the aetiology and treatment of urinary symptoms in women. *British Medical Journal* 294:540-543.

Malouff, J. M., and R. I. Lanyon. 1985. Avoidant paruresis: An exploratory study. *Behavior Modification* 9:225-234.

Margolis, G. J. 1965. A review of literature on psychogenic urinary retention. *Journal of Urology* 94:257-258.

Markway, B. G., C. N. Carmin, C. A. Pollard, and T. Flynn. 1992. *Dying of Embarrassment: Help for Social Anxiety and Phobia*. Oakland, Calif.: New Harbinger.

Marshall, J. R. 1994. *Social Phobia: From Shyness to Stage Fright*. New York: Basic Books.

McCracken, L. M., and K. T. Larkin. 1991. Treatment of paruresis with in vivo desensitization: A case report. *Journal of Behavior Therapy and Experimental Psychology* 22:57-62.

Menninger, K. A. 1941. Some observations on the psychological factors in urination and genito-urinary afflictions. *Psychoanalytic Review* 28:117-129.

Men's Health. 1997. Malegrams: Mind over bladder. October, 40.

Middlemist, R. D., E. S. Knowles, and C. F. Matter. 1976. Personal space invasions in the lavatory: Suggestive evidence of arousal. *Journal of Personality and Social Psychology* 33:541-546.

Montague, D. K., and L. R. Jones. 1979. Psychogenic urinary retention. *Urology* 13:30-35.

Mozdzierz, G. J. 1985. The use of hypnosis and paradox in the treatment of a case of chronic urinary retention/"bashful bladder." *American Journal of Clinical Hypnosis* 28:43-47.

National Institute of Mental Health. 1994. *Anxiety Disorders.* Washington, D.C.: NIMH.

Newman, E. 1997. *Going Abroad.* St. Paul, Minn.: Marlor Press.

Nicolau, R., J. Toro, and C. P. Prado. 1991. Behavioral treatment of a case of psychogenic urinary retention. *Journal of Behavior Therapy and Experimental Psychology* 22:63-68.

Norden, C. W., and E. A. Friedman. 1961. Psychogenic urinary retention: Report of two cases. *New England Journal of Medicine* 264:1096-1097.

Ost, L. G. 1987. Applied relaxation: Description of a coping technique and review of controlled studies. *Behaviour Research and Therapy.* 26: 13–22

Palmtag, H., and G. Riedasch. 1980. Psychogenic voiding patterns. *Urologia Internationalis* 35:321-327.

Pathak, B. 1995. History of toilets. Paper presented at the International Symposium on Public Toilets, May, 25–27 in Hong Kong.

Pedersen, V. C. 1923. Retention neurosis of the bladder, secondary to postoperative catheterization. *New York Medical Journal and Medical Record* 118:269-272.

Ray, I., and J. Morphy. 1975. Metronome conditioned relaxation and urinary retention. *Canadian Psychiatric Association Journal* 20:139-141.

Rees, B., and D. Leach. 1975. The social inhibition of micturition paruresis: Sex similarities and differences. *Journal of the American College Health Association* 23:203-205.

Ritch, C. O. 1946. Urologic neurosis and psychoses. *Illinois Medical Journal* 89:131-132.

Rosario, D. J., C. R. Chapple, P. R. Tophill, and H. H. Woo. 2000. Urodynamic assessment of the bashful bladder. *Journal of Urology* 163:215-220.

Scott, F. B., E. M. Quesada, and D. Cardus. 1961. Studies on the dynamics of micturition: Observations of healthy men. *Journal of Urology* 92:455-463.

Seif, B. 1982. Hypnosis in a man with fear of voiding in public facilities. *American Journal of Clinical Hypnosis* 24:288-289.

Shatinsky, D., technical advisor for the Secretary of the U.S. Department of Transportation, Drug and Alcohol Policy Office. Conversation with author, September 15, 1999.

Silverman, P. 1980. *Mutual Help Groups: Organization and Development.* Beverly Hills, Calif.: Sage.

Stams, U. K., C. H. Martin, and T. G. Tan. 1982. Psychogenic urinary retention in an eight-year-old boy. *Urology* 20:83-85.

Stanton, S. 1976. Urinary retention in women. *British Medical Journal* (August 14):420-421.

Tanagho, E. A., and E. R. Miller. 1970. Initiation of voiding. *British Journal of Urology* 42:175-183.

Thyer, B. A., and G. C. Curtis. 1984. Furosemide as an adjunct to exposure therapy of psychogenic urinary retention. *Perceptual and Motor Skills* 59:114.

Urinary retention in women. 1976. *British Medical Journal* (June 26):1554.

Van der Linden, E. F., and P. L. Venema. 1998. Acute urinary retention in women. *Ned Tijdschr Geneeskd* 142:1603-1606.

Wahl, C. W., and J. S. Golden. 1963. Psychogenic urinary retention: Report of 6 cases. *Psychosomatic Medicine* 25:543-555.

Weissberg, J. H., and A. N. Levay. 1979. Difficulty in urinating in public rest rooms. *Patient Care* (April): 1–4.

Williams, G. E., and A. M. Johnson. 1956. Recurrent urinary retention due to emotional factors: Report of a case. *Psychosomatic Medicine* 28:77-80.

Williams, G. W., and E. T. Degenhardt. 1954. Paruresis: A survey of a disorder of micturition. *Journal of General Psychology* 51:19-29.

Willimon, W. 1994. Battling bashful bladder syndrome, *USA Today,* October 13.

Wilson, G. T. 1973. Case reports and studies: Innovations in the modification of phobic behaviors in two clinical cases. *Behavior Therapy* 4:426-430.

Winsbury-White, H. P. 1936. Two cases of retention of urine in women. *The Lancet* (May 2):1008-1009.

Wobus, R. E. 1922. Notes on the psychic influence on bladder disturbances in women. *Journal of the Missouri State Medical Association* 19:111-113.

Zgourides, G. D. 1987. Paruresis: Overview and implications for treatment. *Psychological Reports* 60:1171-1176.

———. 1988. Bethanechol chloride as a suggested adjunct to prolonged in vivo exposure therapy in the treatment of paruresis. *Perceptual and Motor Skills* 66:319-322.

———. 1991. Atenolol treatment of paruresis. *Psychological Reports* 68:766.

———. 1996. Management of paruresis by urinary self-catheterization. *Anxiety Disorder Practice Journal* 2:197-198.

Zgourides, G. D., and R. Warren. 1990. Propranolol treatment of paruresis psychogenic urinary retention: A brief case report. *Perceptual and Motor Skills* 71:885-886.

Zgourides, G. D., R. Warren, and M. Englert. 1990. Use of a portable radio headset as an adjunct to exposure therapy in treating paruresis. *Phobia Practice and Research Journal* 3:43-44.

Steven Soifer, M.S.W., Ph.D., is President and Cofounder of the International Paruresis Association and a recovering paruretic. He conducts workshops around the world to help others who suffer from paruresis. He is also Associate Professor at University of Maryland School of Social Work.

George D. Zgourides, Psy.D., is the foremost academic expert on paruresis and has written numerous peer-reviewed journal articles on the subject. He is a clinical psychologist who has specialized in treating this problem and other anxiety disorders. He is also an adjunct faculty member at the Harold Abel School of Psychology at Capella University in Minneapolis, Minnesota.

Joseph Himle, M.S.W., Ph.D., has extensive experience in treating paruretics and developed a treatment manual on which this book is based. He is Associate Director of the Anxiety Disorders Program and Assistant Clinical Professor at the University of Michigan Department of Psychiatry.

Nancy L. Pickering has served as a board member for the International Paruresis Association for two years and is currently serving as Secretary of the organization. She is a published author in the medical and spiritual fields.

Some Other New Harbinger Self-Help Titles

Family Guide to Emotional Wellness, $24.95
Undefended Love, $13.95
The Great Big Book of Hope, $15.95
Don't Leave it to Chance, $13.95
Emotional Claustrophobia, $12.95
The Relaxation & Stress Reduction Workbook, Fifth Edition, $19.95
The Loneliness Workbook, $14.95
Thriving with Your Autoimmune Disorder, $16.95
Illness and the Art of Creative Self-Expression, $13.95
The Interstitial Cystitis Survival Guide, $14.95
Outbreak Alert, $15.95
Don't Let Your Mind Stunt Your Growth, $10.95
Energy Tapping, $14.95
Under Her Wing, $13.95
Self-Esteem, Third Edition, $15.95
Women's Sexualitites, $15.95
Knee Pain, $14.95
Helping Your Anxious Child, $12.95
Breaking the Bonds of Irritable Bowel Syndrome, $14.95
Multiple Chemical Sensitivity: A Survival Guide, $16.95
Dancing Naked, $14.95
Why Are We Still Fighting, $15.95
From Sabotage to Success, $14.95
Parkinson's Disease and the Art of Moving, $15.95
A Survivor's Guide to Breast Cancer, $13.95
Men, Women, and Prostate Cancer, $15.95
Make Every Session Count: Getting the Most Out of Your Brief Therapy, $10.95
Virtual Addiction, $12.95
After the Breakup, $13.95
Why Can't I Be the Parent I Want to Be?, $12.95
The Secret Message of Shame, $13.95
The OCD Workbook, $18.95
Tapping Your Inner Strength, $13.95
Binge No More, $14.95
When to Forgive, $12.95
Practical Dreaming, $12.95
Healthy Baby, Toxic World, $15.95
Making Hope Happen, $14.95
I'll Take Care of You, $12.95
Survivor Guilt, $14.95
Children Changed by Trauma, $13.95
Understanding Your Child's Sexual Behavior, $12.95
The Self-Esteem Companion, $10.95
The Gay and Lesbian Self-Esteem Book, $13.95
Making the Big Move, $13.95
How to Survive and Thrive in an Empty Nest, $13.95
Living Well with a Hidden Disability, $15.95
Overcoming Repetitive Motion Injuries the Rossiter Way, $15.95
What to Tell the Kids About Your Divorce, $13.95
The Divorce Book, Second Edition, $15.95
Claiming Your Creative Self: True Stories from the Everyday Lives of Women, $15.95
Taking Control of TMJ, $13.95
Winning Against Relapse: A Workbook of Action Plans for Recurring Health and Emotional Problems, $14.95
Facing 30: Women Talk About Constructing a Real Life and Other Scary Rites of Passage, $12.95
The Worry Control Workbook, $15.95
Wanting What You Have: A Self-Discovery Workbook, $18.95
When Perfect Isn't Good Enough: Strategies for Coping with Perfectionism, $13.95
Earning Your Own Respect: A Handbook of Personal Responsibility, $12.95
High on Stress: A Woman's Guide to Optimizing the Stress in Her Life, $13.95
Infidelity: A Survival Guide, $13.95
Stop Walking on Eggshells, $14.95
Consumer's Guide to Psychiatric Drugs, $16.95
The Fibromyalgia Advocate: Getting the Support You Need to Cope with Fibromyalgia and Myofascial Pain, $18.95
Working Anger: Preventing and Resolving Conflict on the Job, $12.95
Healthy Living with Diabetes, $13.95
Better Boundries: Owning and Treasuring Your Life, $13.95
Goodbye Good Girl, $12.95
Fibromyalgia & Chronic Myofascial Pain Syndrome, $19.95
The Depression Workbook: Living With Depression and Manic Depression, $17.95

Call **toll free, 1-800-748-6273,** or log on to our online bookstore at **www.newharbinger.com** to order. Have your Visa or Mastercard number ready. Or send a check for the titles you want to New Harbinger Publications, Inc., 5674 Shattuck Ave., Oakland, CA 94609. Include $3.80 for the first book and 75¢ for each additional book, to cover shipping and handling. (California residents please include appropriate sales tax.) Allow two to five weeks for delivery.

Prices subject to change without notice.